DATE DUE

OE 1 '97			
NO 5 '99			
AP 15 02			
AG 2 05			
AP 17 06			
FE 8 07			
MY 18 07			
FE 2 3 08			

DEMCO 38-296

G. Cajetan Luna

Youths Living with HIV
Self-Evident Truths

Pre-publication
REVIEWS,
COMMENTARIES,
EVALUATIONS . . .

"**O**ne of the most challenging health issues for the next millenium is the social rupture caused by AIDS. Everyone will have to face this reality and decide how to deal with this basic truth of life and death: a global virus. Will love be the best vaccine? Or will simple sexual lies be the most inexpensive killing weapon? Will teenagers consciously choose between peace or war? Who will be the winner in our daily social battlefield: a healthy or a risky youth?

Luna's book is a key tool for finding some answers for this future gap. His involving descriptions of adolescents living and struggling with HIV and AIDS is a lesson for everyone. He brings up excruciating aspects of the underground world and demystifies all the hypocracy involved with a direct style, crude language, and bodyflesh truths.

The depth of this book is a *must* for all healthcare professionals, people concerned with youths, and anyone who wants to go beyond the known stereotyped facts of the HIV/AIDS pandemic."

Evelyn Eisenstein, MD
Assistant Professor/
Director of Adolescent Services,
University of Rio de Janeiro

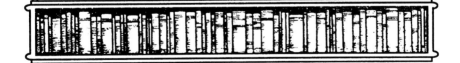

The Haworth Press, Inc.

Youths Living with HIV
Self-Evident Truths

HAWORTH Gay & Lesbian Studies
John P. De Cecco, PhD
Editor in Chief

Youths Living with HIV
Self-Evident Truths

G. Cajetan Luna

The Haworth Press
New York • London

The Haworth Press, Inc., 10 Alice Street, Binghamton, NY 13904-1580

Excerpt from "Days of 1909, 1910, 1911" in *The Complete Poems of Cavafy*, copyright ©1961 and renewed 1989 by Rae Dalven, reprinted by permission of Harcourt Brace & Company.

"I Return for My Wings" from *Poems of Frederica Garcia Lorca*, translated by S Spender and JL Gili. Translation copyright 1939 by S Spender and JL Gili. Used by permission of Oxford University Press, Inc.

The Triumph of Pan by Victor B. Neuburg. Copyright 1989. Reprinted by permission of Skoob Books Publishing Ltd.

"Night Visit" by Tennessee Williams, from *Androgyne, Mon Amour*. Copyright © 1977 by Tennessee Williams. Reprinted by permission of New Directions Publishing Corp.

Cover design by Becky J. Salsgiver.

Library of Congress Cataloging-in-Publication Data

Luna, G. Cajetan.
    Youths living with HIV : self-evident truths / G. Cajetan Luna.
        p.   cm.
    Includes bibliographical references and index.
    ISBN 0-7890-0176-4 (alk. paper)
    1. AIDS (Disease)—United States—Case studies. 2. Young adults—Diseases—United States. I. Title.
RC607.A26L86 1997
382.1'969792'00842—DC21

                                                                                    96-51906
                                                                                    CIP

**FOR MARY ROMERO, MICHAEL H. TROIA,
AND JOSUE INACIO FERREIRA,
THE BEST I HAVE TO GIVE THEM.**

*All the acts and accidents of daily life borrowed a sacred colour and
significance; the very colours of things became themselves weighty with
meanings like the sacred stuffs of Moses' tabernacle, full of penitence or
peace.*

Walter Pater, "The Child in the House," 1895

*Passing all partial loves, this one complete—the mother—
love and sex—emotion blended—
I see the where for centuries thou hast walked,
lonely the world of men,
Saving, redeeming, drawing all to thee,
Yet outcast, slandered, pointed of the mob,
misjudged and crucified.*

Edward Carpenter, "O Child of Uranus," 1912

*I wish for a moment to give sharp attention to the reality of human
happiness in despair: when one is suddenly alone, confronting one's
sudden ruin, when one witnesses the irremediable destruction of one's
work and self. I would give all the wealth of this world—indeed it must
be given—to know the desperate—and secret—state which no one knows
I know.*

Jean Genet, "The Thief's Journal," 1954

ABOUT THE AUTHOR

G. Cajetan Luna is Executive Director of the San Joaquin AIDS Foundation in Stockton, California, and has served as an advisor and consultant to the Pan American Health Organization, Columbia University, UCLA, and UCSF. Mr. Luna's work has been published in a variety of professional journals—his current writing focuses on the challenges facing those living with HIV and AIDS in rural America. He has conducted extensive research with homeless youths in South America and the United States, with long-term and ongoing field study in Rio de Janeiro, Brazil. Mr. Luna's postgraduate work at UCSF and Berkeley was in the fields of medical anthropology, epidemiology, and adolescent health.

CONTENTS

Preface

In the reproof of chance
Lies the true proof of men: The sea being smooth,
How many shallow bauble boats dare sail
Upon her patient breast, making their way
With those of nobler bulk?

–William Shakespeare, *Troilus and Cressida*, 1601-1603

At first this was research. I wrote down silences, nights,
I noted the inexpressible. I fixed vertigos.

–Arthur Rimbaud, *A Season in Hell*, 1939

People live out their biographies from one generation to the next within society, and follow a historical sequence (Mills, 1959). Merely through living, they contribute, however minutely, to shaping their societies and the course of their history, even as they themselves are affected by larger historical patterns and processes. The private "troubles" of individuals and the larger institutional public "issues" of societies are inextricably linked (Mills, 1959). Individuals, societies, and nations are increasingly interdependent. These notions have gained validity and international relevance in the past decade as increases in HIV (human immunodeficiency virus) infections and the ever-growing AIDS (acquired immunodeficiency syndrome) pandemic have globally challenged the resources and abilities of health professionals, public-policy makers, and their respective governments in response. This book addresses one aspect of this much larger problem, focusing on the lives of young people living with HIV. It is hoped that by presenting the private "troubles" and experiences of youths, dependent and larger public "issues" regarding HIV infection and AIDS are identified, and the need for comprehensive and targeted preventative and interventive measures are demonstrated.

The detailed narrative information included in this book was collected by ethnographers of the Joven Project, which started in October 1992 and explored and documented the lives of youth living with HIV and AIDS over a two-year period. This multisite, ethnographic, exploratory study was one component of a larger, National Institute on Drug Abuse (NIDA)-supported Secondary AIDS Education and Prevention Program to reduce HIV risk acts in a broad spectrum of young people in AIDS epicenters in the eastern and western United States. The conceptual framework for the Secondary Prevention Program focused on personal vulnerability, enhanced motivation to act safely, and the acquisition of behavioral skills. An additional goal was to develop reliable and valid assessments of sexual and substance-use risk acts. At the time this program was initiated, little was known about youths living with HIV and AIDS. The Joven Project was conducted in the first stages of the program in order to inform the development of the educational intervention; to generate and reveal themes relevant to program goals; and to illustrate life experiences, challenges, and related lifestyles of the youths.

Interviews were conducted following referrals through collaborating agencies and institutions, and through informal networks of male and female youths and young adults living with HIV or AIDS, ages nineteen to twenty-five, and self-identified as bisexual, gay, heterosexual, or transgendered. All racial groups were included. Anglo and African Americans were overrepresented. Both urban and suburban youth were interviewed. The majority were gay-identified, coupled or single; others were heterosexual, married, and parenting. Many were pursuing higher education; most had high school diplomas or equivalency. Twenty-five were actively or previously involved as peer educators, speakers, and program support staff or facilitators.

Four experienced social scientists, including the author, who was Project Director and Supervisor, and ethnographers Hilarie Kelly, Toby Marotta, and Dorinda Welle conducted the research collaboratively but independently on both coasts of the United States. Over sixty youths were followed in-depth and over time, and an additional eighty-five were interviewed episodically. As Project Director, I had the unique role of not only interviewing and following youths on the West Coast, but reviewing all interviews and transcripts from all sites, identifying patterns in life stories, and discussing evolving themes with ethnographers on a regular basis.

Institutional Review Board (IRB) approval was obtained, and signed consent was given by participants to audiotape interviews. Ethnographers initially followed a protocol so that basic demographic information could be collected and compared. Initial interviews were open-ended, and in subsequent interviews, evolving issues or themes were explored. Most interviews were tape recorded and subsequently transcribed. Health and social service experts were similarly interviewed to determine the extent and quality of service provision during the study period. Along with demographic background and family histories, many other dimensions were explored, including the problems youth encountered on a daily basis, their activities, social networks, adaptational strategies, and coping methods. As the narratives will illustrate, individuals used both socially competent and incompetent ways of coping with their lives and with HIV infection. Social networks and circumstances influenced their activities and behavioral practices. Similarities in the dimensions of lives, and major themes in the natural history of HIV in youths and young adults existed. Four central thematic areas were explored:

- The background that led up to infection, including personal family history and problems, sexual preference, substance abuse behaviors, runaway history, and socioeconomic conditions.
- Their beliefs on how and why their infection occurred, with attention to behavioral mediators, or under what circumstances–when, where, and why–infection occurred, their introduction to risky behaviors, competing risks, their patterns of relationships, and instances of victimization.
- Their experiences associated with the HIV test and notification, including the context and consequences of testing, whether the test was linked with services or anonymous, and whether testing positive was a traumatic or inconsequential experience.
- Their experiences subsequent to testing HIV positive, or the outcomes, with attention to adaptation and coping, disclosure, quality of life, future orientation, and the role of services and providers.

The underlying issues and themes connected to these areas typify characteristics in the common challenge of adaptation to HIV that most youths experienced. Confidentiality was maintained. Data analysis was continuous; similar interviewee statements were compared and categorized. Definitions and meanings of life recollections were examined, and patterns and themes evolved providing additional understanding of the larger social world of youth living with HIV and AIDS (Glaser and Strauss, 1967; Langness and Frank, 1981; Strauss and Corbin, 1990; Brown and Langley, 1991). Personal narratives presented in this volume were constructed from this data. Narratives provide important in-depth and contextual information about how youths achieved order–gaining stability and regulating out-of-control behavior–and obtained meaning from their experiences (Vasina, 1965). Narratives are presented to illustrate the complex efforts these youths made to make sense of threatened lives. This book presents representative and focused narrative case studies, including extensive life recollections of youths living with HIV and AIDS. The cases selected typify the central themes and issues to the entire sample, and reflect the demographic variation. However, those represented here were atypical in important ways. These youths were more verbal and communicative about their lives, were better connected to social or health service agencies, and in all but one instance (Jared), were aware of their HIV infection for more than six months before the interviews started. In addition, the study population on-the-whole faced particular and extraordinary life challenges and dysfunctions. They represent the early instances of HIV infections in youths in the United States–individuals whose life circumstances made them particularly vulnerable. Increasingly, the population of adolescents and young adults living with HIV and AIDS is becoming more diverse, and characteristically is comprised of youths with less problematic familial or social backgrounds. Nevertheless, youths facing serious life challenges and dysfunctions, such as those studied, will likely experience the first wave of future public-health threats. From the experiences recorded and documented, significant predictive, preventive, and interventive lessons can be learned, and these lessons have important future applicability.

I rediscovered Walt Whitman's writings as this study progressed, and they influenced my own cosmology, understanding, and intent.

In the following chapters, this influence will become more evident. For now, it is useful to recollect Whitman's advice not to depict evil and the negative for its own sake. Evil and the negative should not overshadow a work. Instead, as with Shakespeare, *evil was a foil for the positive and the pure.* Whitman encouraged writers to present the more positive aspects of life, "As in some vast foundry whose wells are lost in blackness, a scuttle far up in the roof lets the sun and the blue sky in" (Garland, 1929). This is especially relevant, but difficult for those who describe everyday activities and lives–especially activities and lives with dark, obscure, or tragic dimensions. The hidden meanings that characterize less-visible psychological and social worlds must be sought. Some readers may believe that focusing on the sexual lives and troubles of teenagers in the detail that follows is exploitive. However disconcerting such a focus may be, it is essential to see the interconnected and damaging effects that early–if not coerced–initiation into sexual activity and instances of physical and sexual abuse have on subsequent life development and young adulthood. There is an erroneous tendency to blame the victims, to consider behaviors as irresponsible, and to portray the end result of their actions as somehow deserved. A close reading of the lives that follow will illustrate how inexperience and vulnerability were easily exploited. It is hoped that the reader will discern *positive insights* in the lives presented. These are not works of fiction, wherein control could be exercised over the recollections of the young people presented; nor could an artificial and positive emphasis be given to private troubles or tragic life events. The meanings of these narratives are neither identical nor immediately obvious; they are suggestive. The consequences of a range of mean and demeaning life circumstances, and the meanings youths attached to them are *self-evident.*

This book reconstructs the past and present struggles that young people with HIV and AIDS faced and continue to face. Initially, HIV infection was assumed to play a greater role in their lives than in most instances was actually the case. HIV was significant, but it was not the predominant concern for most youths, after notification. Their life circumstances and social worlds before notification played important roles in how they experienced and responded to their infections. Some youths' significant others included a cast of underworld characters: drug dealers, needle users, pornographers, fetishists, and thieves. Other important people included parents, siblings, extended family, college students, recent immigrants to the United States, individuals with full-time day jobs, and people with no interest in drug use or street culture whatsoever. It must be emphasized that underworld characters also maintained lives in the mainstream society and economy, and friendship groupings often overlapped. The issues that concerned the majority studied were incest, abuse, rape, sexuality or sexual expression, imbalanced relationships, and especially the achievement of respectability and stability. Life challenges and struggles were not characteristically HIV-related, but were more closely tied to past or present experiences of emotional abandonment; broken trust; poverty; physical and sexual abuse; discrimination based upon ethnicity, gender, and sexual orientation; and the resulting social and emotional disenfranchisement. The narratives illustrate the insights and dignity of young people confronting less-than-positive life challenges and circumstances. The accompanying discussion attempts to identify and disentangle the major themes. Given difficult past experiences and histories, "simply" to survive and function may seem miraculous for many youths living with HIV and AIDS. However, upon closer examination, the narratives not only reflect larger social and institutional inadequacies, they also demonstrate youths' personal and individual spirit, strength, and resiliency.

Acknowledgments

*Wings, wings! I beheld the young leaves breaking from the buds
and poised on the tips of the branches.*

—Edward Carpenter, "Wings", 1912

The ethnographic interviews that are the basis for this book were conducted primarily with the financial support of the National Institute on Drug Abuse (NIDA) through a multisite grant to Mary Jane Rotheram-Borus, Principal Investigator (#1R01DA07903-01). Some of the case studies included in this volume have been, or will be published in different forms (Rotheram-Borus et al., 1994; Luna and Rotheram-Borus, 1997a,b). I thank the publishers for permission to reprint versions tailored for this volume, including the editors of *NIDA Research Monograph*, Number 143. I acknowledge the significant contributions of Hilarie Kelly (ethnographer, southern West Coast), Robert Payne (Toby) Marotta (ethnographer, northern West Coast), and especially Dorinda Welle (ethnographer, East Coast); the suggestions and revisions of Mary Jane Rotheram-Borus; the editorial work of Lisa J. Franko, Dawn Krisko, Kris Langabeer, and Peg Marr; and the advice of Richard C. Brown, John P. De Cecco, Robert B. Edgerton, Geoffrey Froner, Edward Kuczynski, and the late Anselm L. Strauss. Former teachers and colleagues including Joan Ablon, Lydia S. Bond, Margaret Clark, Nicolette Collins, Evelyn Eisenstein, Diane Flannery, Evelyn S. Gendel, and Karen Heller have provided valuable insights and perspectives on marginalized youths. Financial and personal support for the writing of this book came from Patrick Alexon, Hilario Luna, Marie and Ted Teach, and Jeffrey Terrell. This book would not have been completed without their patient and persistent encouragement. I hope my colleagues, friends, and family take as their influence those parts that please them and forgive me the rest. The analysis and conclusions are mine alone and are not necessarily opinions shared by these or other associates. Institutional and clerical support was given at different periods by the University of California, the HIV Center of Columbia University, the State University of Rio de Janeiro (UERJ), Brazil, and the Pan American Health Organization, Regional Office of the World Health Organization. University-affiliated health clinics and community-based social service agencies provided access to youths and were critical to this research. The contributions of young people living in the eastern and western United States whose lives are described in this book are most sincerely appreciated–*di uortant bene.*

Portland, Oregon

Chapter 1

Introduction

*For these associations originating outside, and
these borrowed emotions, carry young people over
the dangerously soft spiritual ground of the years in
which they need to be of some significance to themselves and nevertheless are still too incomplete to
have any real significance. Whether any residue of
it is ultimately left in the one, or nothing in the
other, does not matter; later each will somehow
come to terms with himself (herself), and the danger exists only in the stage of transition.*

–Robert Musil, *Young Torless*, 1955

In the United States of the early 1980s, AIDS affected primarily
white, urban, male homosexuals between the ages of twenty-five
and forty-five with histories of multiple sexual activities with
strangers (Fremont-Smith, 1983). By the close of the decade,
females, heterosexuals, youths, and those of all races who were
sexually abstinent and had undergone blood transfusions or shared
infected needles were understood to be at risk based upon their
activities or behaviors (Bond, 1992). The false sense of security
held by Americans about who was infected and where they lived
began to erode. HIV infections spread beyond the initial risk groups
of homosexual men, intravenous drug users, and hemophiliacs
(Poppen and Reisen, 1994).

Reflecting these demographics, AIDS health services and prevention programs were initially developed and located in more pop-
ulous, heterogeneous urban cities and served mostly adult, gay male
populations. By the late 1980s service programs for youths and
females became more commonplace. Attention was increasingly

focused on prevention and intervention with urban and suburban male and female high school students, youths entering military services, and eventually on poor or homeless youths living with HIV and AIDS (Luna, 1987a; Luna, 1991; Luna and Rotheram-Borus, 1992). Initially, there was a tendency to represent youths living with HIV and AIDS as a special interest group, a class, a cause. Considering them like other "risk groups" depersonalized their particular circumstances and dehumanized their individual plights. Their private struggles and troubles, as well as their personal accomplishments were minimized. Research both preceded and accompanied service interventions for high-risk and in-school youths. However, research rarely concentrated on the range of experiences of youths living with HIV (Luna, Bond, and Zacarias, 1992). Research focused even less upon the circumstances, experiences, and lives of gay-identified, middle-class, or not-homeless youths living with HIV.

The lives of young males and females who self-identify as homosexual or gay can be particularly challenging regardless of their economic class or place of residence (Martin and Hetrick, 1988). Youths who act upon their sexual preference are often the victims of ridicule and physical abuse. During their childhood and adolescence, many of these young people do not have the developmentally linked skills to combat the labels that are attached to them. When they identify and meet "comrades in nature," they are often adults and not peers. Gay-identified youths are unconnected to larger reference groups that could provide them with objective help. They are unaware of other prominent people who have shared their sexual preference (Ellis and Symonds, 1897; Rowse, 1977; Dover, 1978; Sarotte, 1978) and as a result, lack identifiable and positive role models (Leyland, 1978; Leyland, 1982). With few opportunities for contact with same-preference peers (if desired), males in particular often engage in cross-generational, power-imbalanced, same-sex relationships and fail to make self-protective decisions during sexual activities (Luna, 1994b).

When homosexual young people inform others of their sexual preference, there are often repercussions (Martin and Hetrick, 1988). The process of *coming out* occurs when they frankly present themselves to family, friends, or co-workers as homosexual, or *gay* (Hooker, 1956; Hunter and Schaecher, 1994). Often accomplished through public demonstrations or as a personally relevant *rite of passage*, coming out is a difficult and stressful process, especially for youths who are not legally emancipated. Parental responses range from acceptance and approval to rejection and total abandonment. The latter response is more frequent. Coming out as homosexual often has less consequence than coming out as HIV positive. Youths who hide their sexual orientation from family, friends, or co-workers, and live *closeted*, frequently choose to come out as homosexual and HIV positive simultaneously. As a result, their problems are compounded, especially if they live in communities that do not support social and sexual diversity.

Young heterosexual males or females living with HIV and AIDS also experience significant problems after infection. Many support services for gay-identified people living with HIV and AIDS have been established within gay communities. However, fewer exist that are tailored to the specific needs of heterosexuals in the same circumstances. The stigma attached to risk behaviors (including anal intercourse) and risk groups (including homosexuals and intravenous drug users) leads many young heterosexuals living with HIV and AIDS to hide their health status from family, friends, or even sexual partners. Those who do disclose to partners face abandonment or physical and emotional abuse. Those who disclose to family face being ostracized, and they often experience discrimination such as eviction from housing and barriers within the public education system. Thus, heterosexuals who come out as HIV infected face similar problems as youths coming out as gay. Heterosexual and homosexual youths of color living with HIV face additional challenges within families, communities, and the health care system. They have problems accessing services relevant to their particular cultural experiences and identities. Problems, tensions, and mistrust exists across racial, ethnic, and gender lines. Those who are uncomfortable in gay-oriented settings are particularly reluctant to attend programs at gay-identified agencies and often do not take advantage of therapeutic treatments or support services of potential benefit. Young women who, as a result of pregnancy, learn of their HIV infection or subsequent to their infection decide to have children often are faced with serious decisions including abortion, adoption, and child care should they become incapacitated or if their death becomes more imminent.

The lives of adolescents and young adults living with HIV and AIDS studied were not simple. In addition to AIDS-related concerns, there were normal developmental and maturational challenges of separation and sexual-identity formation, and self-doubts concerning personal abilities and appropriate behaviors in oftentimes perplexing settings or situations. The transition between late adolescence and young adulthood requires adaptations and adjustments to physical, physiological, psychological, sexual, and social role changes. For most, this period is relatively easy and may represent the best years in the life cycle. For those challenged by a life-threatening illness, this period is more difficult, as normal developmental stressors and problems are compounded by accompanying disease-related experiences. These experiences can facilitate continued or increased alienation and self-harmful behaviors. They can also prove motivational, forcing actions to be taken, offering new hope, or giving future direction to life plans. The following narratives of youths living with HIV illustrate both.

Chapter 2

"Famous Runaway": Jose

Then down the forest aisles there came a boy,
Unearthly pale, with passion in his eye;
Who sang a song whereof the sound was joy,
But all the burden was of love that dies
And death that lives—a song of sobs and sighs,
A wild swan's note of Death and Love in one.

—John Addington Symonds, *Tema con Variazioni*, 1878

Jose was an animated and energetic twenty-three-year-old Latino. He self-identified as gay although he disliked labels. He was the oldest of four children born in the eastern United States. His father worked in a candy factory, and Jose clearly remembered giving away "bags and bags of candy" to other children to make them like him. He was still trying "to lose the weight from eighth grade." His mother also worked, and in early childhood, he was raised by his maternal grandmother in Latin America. During his early adolescence he had daily confrontations with his father, who strongly disapproved of Jose's "less-than-masculine" appearance. He angrily recalled that his father ridiculed his aspirations to be an artist and compared his father to a 1970s television sitcom character: "He's like Mr. Brady on drugs."

> I grew up with my dad having a six-pack of beer and a pint of Jack Daniels for breakfast—that looked so normal, growing up. . . . I thought that every man was supposed to hit their wife and drink. I thought that was a man's job.

Jose failed most of his courses in high school, although he excelled in drama classes, where he remembers being able to "become everybody else except myself." He left before graduating and fantasized about going back to his high school a success.

> I always think that maybe I'll become rich and famous. Then they'll understand. I'll go to a class reunion where I never really graduated, but I'll go with some friend who graduated from there, and I'm going to say, "Oh, you guys stayed in school? What you're pregnant? Ha-Ha-Ha. Look at the millions I have." . . . I've got six years to become rich and famous.

He ran away from home for the first time at age fifteen, taking a bus to the West Coast, hoping to fulfill his fantasy in Southern California. He was alone and homeless, and sought help at a youth shelter. To his dismay, the shelter staff's plan was to send him back to his family. He protested, saying that he would be beaten by his father. He even attempted suicide, but was sent home anyway. He ran away a second time the following year. After arriving again in Southern California, he immediately called information and asked for any agency that would assist him without returning him home. He was given the number of the National Runaway Hotline, and they in turn referred him to The Agency. The Agency offered a variety of health and social services to street youths and adolescent sex workers. At the time, The Agency was just about to open a youth shelter. Almost immediately according to Jose, he obtained his "fifteen minutes of fame."

> I became, like, a *famous runaway* when the shelter was open and my picture was on the front of the newspaper. How stupid, huh? I'm a runaway, and I'm on the front of the newspaper. . . . me, walking, fresh, sixteen years old, talking about my dreams and how I came here, and then it's like the end. I mean when the end is coming, I knew I had to say something really catchy. . . . I'm a famous runaway, ha, ha, ha. Let me say something catchy. And I said something like, "I grabbed my star, and I'm not going to let go." Oh gee.

Jose never spoke with his father after he left home, although he maintained contact with other family members, including his mother, whom he telephoned regularly. He recalled that the only time in his life he felt happy and safe was when he was with his mother. Since leaving home, he lived in many places. His drug use history included a variety of substances beginning with alcohol and then progressing to marijuana, cocaine, crack cocaine, and ultimately methamphetamine, or "speed," which he injected using shared needles. His drug use experiences provided him with a rare perspective on suburban life.

> Cocaine, crack, everything except heroin. Crystal meth, I shot up three times. Crystal meth, pot—it's boring though. It just makes you sleepy and tired; all you want to do is eat and go to sleep. With crystal, you don't eat for days. Talk about a great way to diet. Forget Jenny Craig, just shoot up crystal. . . . Have a couple of lines before a meal, forget the Slimfast shake. Just drink that and a beer; believe me, you'll lose the weight. You'll run around your room cleaning everything in sight. A vacuum cleaner couldn't clean better than a person on speed— that's for sure. Gosh, but then the five days afterward are depression, loneliness, oh! Everybody in the world could love you to death, but you still feel the same way. . . . Gives you the greatest rush, but then when you come down—what goes up that high, comes down that low.

He was involved in *street life* after running away, but he would not directly discuss his previous activities, including sex work. However, in criticizing religious conservatives, he provided insight into his past. "They talk about sex, and then they pick up little boys. I know; I went with a minister." Although he had sexual relations with men as far back as his early adolescence, he never established an extended relationship with a particular lover.

Jose believed he contracted HIV through shared intravenous drug use. He recalls being picked up in a gay bar by a slightly older man—"blond, hip, and middle class"—the type he liked. They went to a hotel and had sex. Jose was under the influence of alcohol and orally digested methamphetamine. His sexual partner urged him to inject methamphetamine with him, and Jose agreed even though he had never done so before. The experience was intense, but fleeting. He never saw the blond man again. The next morning he was deeply depressed and cried, fearing the possible consequences of the risk he had taken. Although at the time he believed he might have contracted HIV, he did not test for the virus for more than a year, and he "shot up" on two other occasions with sexual partners. He tested positive in late 1990. He adjusted to his HIV status easier than many others do since he was already a client of the social service system by the time of his infection. His attitude about HIV and AIDS softened over time, as he emphasized, "I said this would never happen to me, and if it does, I'll kill myself–things change."

At age twenty-two, Jose decided "enough was enough," and began to work on his substance abuse problems. He attended both Alcoholics Anonymous (AA) and Narcotics Anonymous (NA) groups. He had occasional relapses and drug binges that complicated getting his life in order. These occurred when his loneliness was especially hard to bear. During these relapses, he generally spent a good deal of money, lost independent housing arrangements, and relied on social service agencies. He carried the burden and stigma of having been a runaway, but nevertheless clung to this part of his past because he believed it made him special. Being a "famous runaway" generated considerable attention for him that was both positive and negative.

Jose's work with agencies gave him a temporary sense of self-esteem and purpose. He had "been through everything," and felt he could relate well with younger, less experienced youths. He worked in both volunteer and paid jobs for The Agency, after having been their client. First, he was their spokesman, and he represented The Agency in public forums both locally and nationally, as well as on television and radio. Subsequently, in a paid job, he did reception work and provided referrals, peer counseling, and public speaking. On a typical workday, he rose at 7:00 a.m. to take the bus to work and did not return home until after 5:00 p.m. However, having a salaried job as a peer educator and a daily routine to follow did not change his chronic cycle of emotional ups and downs. He still had frequent emotional crises, and he would self-medicate his problems through heavy and continuous substance use. In time, and after his role had changed from client to provider, he felt he could not receive the same assistance he had in the past from his female counselor at The Agency.

Well, it isn't the same. It's not the same as it used to be. She isn't the same. . . . Well, I work there, so I can't really call on them.

Because of his employment, Jose was not comfortable talking about his personal problems with the staff at The Agency. He had been dependent upon The Agency for emotional support for years. The Agency now had job-related expectations of him as their employee, that were separate from his own personal and emotional needs as their former client and a young person living with HIV. He was expected to be more self-directed, together, and capable. He believed staff members were not happy to see him fall back into old patterns, and he felt they were less willing to extend him support at this time in his life. There was little or no privacy related to his past problems; everyone at work knew his past history. He was expected to function as an equal with people who knew his past life difficulties but did not reveal their own.

Jose was also a contract employee at the health clinic where he received his HIV-related health services. He was uneasy setting a fee for his services for fear that he might offend or damage a relationship on which he was dependent. His continuing need for medical and psychological services after his positive HIV diagnosis made his work relationships difficult.

Jose feared that when he turned twenty-four and by Agency definition was no longer considered a youth, he would lose eligibility for many of the services he had grown accustomed to since his days as a runaway. He felt increasingly tired and run down and was concerned about his health. He was very attuned to when physical changes occurred in his body. He became depressed when he thought his body was "going down." He was frequently beset by intense feelings of loneliness, which he tried to minimize by spending time with friends, none of whom were living with HIV. He specifically sought friends who were sober, and not substance users. His mood shifted from exuberance, when he fantasized an extravagant future, to deep depression, which occurred when he appraised his current state of affairs: "I'm not going to die unhappy like this, am I?"

On a trip home, he told family members that he was living with HIV. His mother cried at first. "I didn't cry," said Jose, "I took the opportunity to educate her about it." Disclosing his status to his family and educating them about HIV provided the opportunity for family members to help each other. They discussed his HIV and his contingency plan to come home to live with his mother if or when his health declined. However, for the time being, he was going on with his life and not allowing HIV infection to change his life plans.

Jose had lived for a long time in youth shelters, but eventually moved into his own apartment. He lost his job at The Agency because he did not meet their expectations by completely ending his drug use. He was angry and scared about being unemployed. Emotionally, Jose was very vulnerable and dependent, having been an Agency favorite for years. He had been a quasi-celebrity and had been exploited for his early life difficulties. In his midtwenties, unemployed, and living with HIV, he was not the vulnerable teenager or adult success story that could be employed for publicity or fund-raising purposes. He was expendable, like commodities past their use.

Chapter 3

"All These Personal Stories": Jack

Build for yourself but a single nest in a single tree,
such that thither no dangerous creeping beast may climb.
For now you perch one day upon one branch, and next day
Flit to another, always in search of something new.

Do not forget this truth, we were younger a year ago,
and no charm may we find that shall save us from growing old
And wrinkled, nor are we able to capture youth again,
Once it has flown, for the shoulders of youth are fledged with wings,
and we are too slow to catch a creature of flight so swift.

—Theocritus, *Idyll XXIX* (In Trevelyan, 1925)

While Jose was dependent upon service agencies for most of his adolescence and young adulthood, Jack used social services only after his HIV infection was diagnosed. Jack was a bright, articulate, twenty-one-year-old, white, gay male, born in Northeastern United States. He appeared much younger than his age. He spoke quickly and in a nervous, dramatic way. He dressed conservatively, usually in pastel colors, and wore his hair in a neat, short, cropped style. His parents divorced when he was in his early teens. He walked with a slight limp that he attributed to severe anal warts. He had a long history of sexually transmitted diseases (STDs) back to his middle adolescence. During his teens, Jack and his mother (who Jack described as lesbian) moved to the Southeast where he finished high school and met his first lover. He described his first sexual experience in detail, illustrating his independence, and the risks he took early in life.

I was in the grocery store with my mother and she was looking for a lady, and there was this guy there. He was

11

twenty-four at the time, and an actor. . . . My mother put the milk and everything on the counter, and he was looking at me. How am I going to get around this?. . . . I know that I am gay and I know that I have these feelings–I liked the guy–what's it all about? So I grabbed the milk from my mother and said, "Oh, the date on the milk is bad," and I ran and I put it back, and I grabbed another milk. I met the guy and shook hands. He had already written down his name and telephone number. "Give me a call when you get the chance." I did so. She [his mother] went to the laundry the following day. We had to be on the phone a long time because I remember hanging up the moment my mother came walking through the door. He was telling me all these other things, and asking me things, "Do you like to do this?" And all the time I had never done it before, so I told him "Yes. Yes." A lot of those things for the first time seemed a little far-out, but I was thinking about how they would be done, and if he would do them, or if I would do them. It just seemed fun, like, "Wow! Sure." And I remember one day, going over to his house directly after school, telling my mother that I was going to a friend's house. . . . and he gave me an orange juice or something–it was a kid's drink. I was sixteen at the time, and he was twenty-four. I was sitting on the couch and he held my hand and he took me into the bedroom. . . . It did not hurt; I was like, "Wow! this is neat. I like this." . . . I was the one who was taken.

Jack, could not recall the man's name, but remembered that he saw him for a short period. He recalled that the man had gone to the doctor and was told he had the "clap." In hindsight, Jack recognized that "at least the man was honest" in informing him of the doctor's report.

Jack lived with his mother until he could no longer tolerate her alcoholism or continue to "take care of her."

We lived over a bar, and my mom was drinking, I mean drinking severely and totally drunk, hardly could stand up, barely could talk. . . . I was only ten years old. I mean I was really an adult. . . . I was always having to take care of my mother whenever she was drunk. I remember one time dragging her with every bit of energy I had up three flights of stairs, just to bathe her because she would urinate in her pants.

Jack's mother frequently beat him and pulled him down the street by his ears. When problems at home were particularly difficult, he would sleep in public parks. During his early teens, he experimented with sex for money to "see what it was like." Jack went to the shipyards with a "straight" adolescent friend who stayed overnight at his house.

> Well we went down to the shipyards and said, "Whoever wants to take me takes you, too. You know it's a three-way thing and whatever we make we split." Well, this guy drives up in a red truck and he points to me and he said, "Come here." And I went over and he said, "Do you want the job or not?" I knew what he wanted, of course. Because that's the reason we were out there. So I said, "My friend is going, too." He said, "No, only you or nothing." So I went with him. I told my friend, "Wait for me here. I don't care where you go or who picks you up, just come back and wait for me." I went off with the guy and did what I had to. I ended up giving him a blow job and he gave me–I'm embarrassed–I think I got forty dollars. Right after that I got picked up by a guy in a limousine, or a Cadillac. He said, "Get in," and this other kid gets out. And I didn't know where my friend had gone so we were driving around. He just wanted a young kid in the car to masturbate over him. He did what he had to and he ended up giving me twenty dollars, plus finding my friend and feeding us. When he left, I swore I would never do that again. And I never did. So it was a one time thing, wondering what the whole thing was, what it was like.

Jack was sexually active throughout high school, and he moved in with Philip before graduation. Philip was handsome and "butch," about the same age as Jack, and had dropped out of high school. Philip came from a family involved in gangs and organized crime. The two worked menial jobs to pay their rent, and they often found themselves homeless.

We were sleeping in parks. I was sleeping, but I remember waking up to someone pulling on my zipper, and Philip was so exhausted from trying to keep me safe that he passed out; he just wouldn't wake up. This guy started going in my pants and everything, as if I would let him, and I'm thinking, "This guy is raping me." So the only way to stop him was to kick him between his legs, and I kept kicking and kicking and finally Philip woke up. . . . And when Philip woke up and this guy noticed how huge Philip was, this guy left.

His relationship with Philip was short term, and Jack soon entered an alternative high school for gay youth. As he remembers, at the time he was "really getting involved with reading and trying to establish relationships with other males." Subsequently, Jack shared apartments with many "boyfriends." He had verbal and physical altercations with most of his partners. Following these incidents, he would often spend the night in public parks. Jack was tested for HIV at his former Northeast hometown after his physician, who was from the Southeast, refused to test him, thinking Jack was suicidal. He tested positive, and believed he was infected by his first sexual partner.

Like Jose, Jack had been a client of various social service programs for five years. He volunteered as a peer counselor at a medical clinic where he received HIV-related services. He referred to his female social worker as "my only family, my professional mom." He no longer had any contact with either of his biological parents. In the past, he participated in various paid or volunteer HIV forums, and had given local and national media interviews on HIV and AIDS. Jack completed his first year of college, and he planned to get a bachelor's degree in social work to "become a professional peer counselor." He spoke about HIV and AIDS at many locations. In public speaking and through sharing his life story, Jack often elicited emotional reactions from his student audience members who then shared their stories about other people living with AIDS.

Central High had been a sort of place where I felt welcomed. . . . The kids loved me; the teachers loved me. They wanted me there to speak; they wanted to hear what I had to say. There, I even had kids cry in the classrooms and tell me,

"My mother has AIDS," "My mother and father are HIV infected," "I'm sick; I'm dying from AIDS." All the personal things they are telling me, and there are a lot of them. *That* is a school!

Jack emphasized that, in some school districts "you have to be more careful," and that certain audiences are more homophobic than others. Given these circumstances, he believed that he had to sometimes lie about his sexual preference. Jack hid his gay identity during presentations by explaining to his audiences that he had been infected through heterosexual intercourse. He oftentimes could not represent his true sexual preference, his "true self." He believed that his fabricated explanation garnered him "more respect" with audiences, and as a result, the students "liked him more." He described how he explained his HIV infection and the students' response.

This is the first time I had sex, and I was infected with it from that same girl. But, I did tell them I had a lot of sex. They were just, "Oh, you got it from a girl; you know, I can get it from a girl." . . . By telling them that, it made them respect me a little, you know, they said, "I like this boy; I like this guy."

As intended, the peer educator role provided Jack the opportunity to speak to other students, and to relate and share experiences with them. However, he also became more aware of his own feelings of inadequacy about his past life events and insecurities about whether he would be accepted by peers, many of whom held negative attitudes about his sexual preference. Jack described one incident that was particularly problematic. He engaged in sexual activity with a student he met following an HIV educational presentation at a high school. It was his practice to give students his home address and to offer to answer any unresolved questions or concerns. He described what happened next, and illustrated the difficulty some adolescents experience in juggling roles of educator and sexual being.

Through that school, I met this one kid who wrote me a letter saying, "I don't know if you remember me." I gave the kids my address and said, "Sure, if you have any questions or want someone to talk to, just write me." So this one kid contacts me. He's fifteen years old. I think he was fourteen saying he was going on fifteen, but he said he was fifteen. He wrote me a letter, and he said he would like to talk to me about whatever.

The initial contact through the mail developed into a face-to-face meeting. Jack initially described what happened in the following:

> I kind of thought immediately, he didn't state the issue—underlying issue—he didn't state in any way he was gay or that he had friends that were gay, but I just knew that for some reason, he had a feeling for me. And I was sort of turned on. I was very flattered. This was the first time it had ever happened to him. . . . I ended up telling him, "Yes, I do want to have sex with you," after a whole day trying to get it out of him or trying to assure him that it would be okay if he did tell me. He knew that I was HIV positive anyway, after my going to his school. . . . He came to my house. . . . kissed me, and we leaned against each other; it was really nice. There were no fluids being passed; he knew I was HIV positive. It was more. He knew I was HIV positive, and neither one of us wanted to put him at risk, so we just masturbated.

In a follow-up interview, Jack recalled that they did more than just masturbate, "We had full sex, to the point of using a condom." Jack stated that they continued to get together periodically, during which time Jack said they had unsafe sex. He emphasized that the "kid" was aware of the risk he was taking because he knew Jack was infected. Jack also emphasized that "besides, it takes several contacts to transmit HIV to a person." They saw each other a few months. He believed the chances of the fifteen-year-old getting infected were "slim."

> You know he called me back a year later to tell me he had a girlfriend and he just did that to. . . He had a girlfriend. Ha ha, *all these personal stories.*

Jack recalled other times when he did not use condoms during sexual activity. He did not feel that he had to self-consciously "manage" his comments during interviews as when he was doing his peer education work, "We didn't use condoms all the time when he was having intercourse with me. . . . It is good to be open." Jack's social worker was aware that he frequently did not tell his sexual partners of his HIV status. His social worker confronted him about the contradiction of doing HIV educational work and not consistently using precautions in his own sexual activities.

> Her thing was, "I don't think you should be getting into peer performances if you are going to get into this behavior." . . . and I said exactly what she wanted to hear, which was, "Fine!"

Contradictions between what was expected of Jack as a peer educator and his own personal behaviors and activities were not resolved within group discussions or meetings of the participants in the peer education program. However, these contradictions were discussed in individual sessions between Jack and his social worker. He was expert at impression management, and could manage appropriate behaviors when needed. He struggled with the belief that people living with HIV should inform their sexual partners about their status and whether those living with HIV should even practice "safer sex."

> I sort of decided if I am going to deal with these people as an educator, if you want to have sex with me after that statement, you know, being HIV positive. . . . Well, I decided most recently, within the last year and a half or so, I wouldn't be such a peer educator and talk about condoms—"You should use them." I should be doing it myself instead of just talking about it. I'm not going to play games anymore, you know. I don't think it's worth it.

The motivation behind peer education programs is to value the experience of youths living with HIV or AIDS and give them the opportunity to share these experiences with others. However, adolescent or young-adult peer educators like Jack found it difficult to maintain a professional role and identity as they faced their own developmental challenges and behavioral dilemmas and contradictions. They often felt devalued as they confronted homophobia, racism, sexism, and other negative attitudes in their groups or audiences. Homophobia in his audiences was a major worry for Jack.

During the course of the interviews, a friend of Jack's, concerned that she had not heard from him in months and after telephoning him repeatedly without success, contacted his landlord. With concern, the friend informed the landlord that Jack "had AIDS and might have died." The landlord had police break into Jack's apartment. Jack was home the day of the break-in. A conflict ensued over tenant's rights, including rights to privacy, and within a month, Jack was evicted and homeless.

Economic and social differences play a role in how and why individuals access resources that are available for young people living with HIV and AIDS. Jose had little at his disposal, was in a constant struggle for survival, and was ultimately dependent upon services for financial and social support. Jack had limited savings and economic resources at his disposal, and he was socially isolated. In comparison, Joshua was raised in a more affluent suburban family. He had more resources available. Nevertheless, his problems were as complex as those of both Jose and Jack.

Chapter 4

"Looking for a Friend": Joshua

Have you learn'd lessons only of those who admired you, and
were tender with you, and stood aside for you?
Have you not learn'd great lessons from those who reject you,
and brace themselves against you? or who treat you with
contempt, or dispute the passage with you?

—Walt Whitman, *Stronger Lessons*, 1888

For Joshua, living anonymously with HIV in the suburbs initially was the life he desired. He was white, twenty-four years old, gay, and articulate, and had been living with HIV for five years near a suburban West Coast beach. He was short in stature and had a youthful, carefree appearance. Josh was the youngest of seven children, ranging in age up to forty. He graduated from high school and had one year of college. He was half Swedish and half Greek. His father was a businessman and his mother a homemaker. His parents moved frequently throughout the country during his early childhood, and he was unable to establish many friendships in early adolescence. Substance abuse was a common feature of his teenage years.

> My mother was an alcoholic; she drank more than I would ever drink in a day. Some of my reasons for drinking, I think, classify me as an alcoholic. I wanted to escape, and I used it to build confidence in various ways....And I did drugs. When I was about twenty, I got to a point where I was just hitting a low point; I was just sick and tired of being sick and tired, and at twenty years old, I did not think it was appropriate.

Josh dated girls in his early adolescence, had girlfriends, but the relationships didn't "click" for him. He never engaged in sexual intercourse with these girlfriends. He considered them only as "friends." Josh had his first sexual experience his senior year in high school. This time the sex "clicked."

> I had a sexual experience with a guy in high school a couple of times, and he got really weirded out and he got married and joined the army and moved to Europe. I look forward to our ten-year high school reunion so I will run into him. . . . You know, I made out with girls and stuff like that, but when he and I fooled around, it clicked for me.

Josh started drinking alcohol in high school and went from drinking a little to drinking "a lot very quickly." He drove to "underground" gay clubs in Southern California where the drug ecstasy was easily available. Acid, mushrooms, marijuana, and cocaine were all commonly used in the nightclub scene, and Josh "pretty much went along with it." Ecstasy "became a necessity to make the night."

> They are all a lot of fun. They are mind-altering and they open up your mind. They lessen your inhibitions and all that. But, you know, especially after an extended period of use, I think you can hardly feel it. It really affects your body, and obviously it is not good for you. I mean, after using ecstasy a lot, you wake up really tired and your body is aching and you feel like you were beat up. That's how I would wake up feeling. You know, like someone was just beating my whole body.

He tested for HIV shortly after turning eighteen. His recollections of when and why he tested are typical of similar accounts of other gay men his age.

> Well, I was a young gay male, and I was obviously in a high-risk group, so I figured I would test. I didn't practice unsafe sex or really risky behavior, but knowing what I knew, I just wanted to get tested for myself to make sure that I was healthy and clean. . . . I mean at the time, I wasn't a very educated person. This was about 1986. I think the beginning of 1987 is when I tested because I just moved out here and I

wasn't very clear about things. I just knew that gay men were getting this disease, so I went to get tested. When you go to get tested, they educate you a little. And actually, I realized that I wasn't at risk, but I went ahead and had the test at that point anyway.

At the time, his test results were negative, and he continued substance use and involvement in the underground nightclub scene. At twenty, Josh still lived in his parent's home. However, he spent portions of every day and some nights at the apartment of his first "real" male lover, Brett, who was an older alcoholic. Brett was a member of Alcoholics Anonymous (AA) and encouraged Josh to join. Josh was soon actively involved in their 12-step program. In detail, he described his efforts to achieve social acceptance in AA.

There are some people in the program that should be in the program every night. I think that we are all alike, but we are all very different in ways. I quit, I got sober at twenty-one. I drank for three years. I think I am different than someone who got sober at forty and has been drinking for twenty-five years. Since I quit drinking, I have not had a desire for a drink. There are a lot of people who say one thing and do another; they can stand up and give a speech and sound incredibly healthy, incredibly well, but they are lying. There are people who can read the 12 steps and tell you the traditions and they don't practice it in their lives. . . . I went to straight meetings when I first got sober, but I go to gay meetings now. In the straight meetings, there is a lot of judgment. You know, it is supposed to be unconditional love, but as soon as you turn your back, "Oh Josh over there, oh he's gay," so I just go where I feel comfortable. I have a few friends from AA, and they intermingle with some of my normie friends. A normie as we call them is someone who is not an alcoholic. . . . Most of my friends in AA are older. People my age in AA are scary. They are really promiscuous. I mean, when you give up one addiction, you get another. A lot of guys my age sleep around, and are kind of shallow, and they don't have much sobriety. . . . People don't talk about sex in the meetings. When I first got sober, sober sex is different than when you are drinking. When you are used to having something—when you first get sober, you have more fears about yourself. Like for me, drinking gave me confidence and gave me personality, and for me, drinking made me who I was, and that was not me, because I was really quiet and really reclusive.

As he attempted to address his problems and troubles, his life took a turn for the worse. He recalled the trust he had in Brett, the sexual activity in their relationship, and why he went to get tested for the second time.

Well, we had sex, but just casual, mutual masturbation, pretty much, and we both got tested and we both were negative, and we dated and basically he slept around and I didn't know it. He slept with someone who had AIDS and found out, so he went and got tested. I did not know because he did not share this with me. Brett had tested positive, and at this point we were having unsafe sex because we thought it was safe because we were both negative. . . . We had unprotected oral sex since we both thought we were safe—at least I did—we didn't have safe sex. He tested positive in February, and just for some reason, I decided that year in August—I went down to get tested. He didn't tell me; I just had this feeling. I don't know why—I can't explain it. I just felt like I wanted to get tested.

Josh tested for HIV at a gay and lesbian social- and health-services center. A friend from AA went with him.

He was Brett's best friend, and he had known Brett's status. He had never told me because he didn't know how to say it because Brett had told him not to tell me. He knew. We went down for the test, and he knew what was going to happen.

Josh returned alone for the results two weeks later. His comments illustrate how abuse and deception occur in both personal and professional relationships, and compound stressful life events.

The doctor called me in and said, "Do these two numbers match?" He said, "Well, you tested positive, twice," because when they test you, they have the Eliza and then they do the Blot testing, and if you test negative, they leave it at that because the second test is more expensive. He said, "You have tested positive on both these tests." And he said, "Are you surprised by this? Why?" And I told him I was in a relationship, and he said, "Have you been monogamous?" I mean, he was real judgmental. I was overwhelmed by it. He gave me this card, and he said, "You need to go see a doctor." And that was it, and then he let me go. . . . I went out to my car and I cried. I sat there and cried. I didn't know what to do, and then I went home–I still lived at home. I just cried and I was really upset and I didn't know what to do. Because, I didn't know who I could tell. I couldn't tell any of my friends. All I kept thinking was that I could not tell anybody this–that is all I kept thinking. And how could I tell Brett because I didn't know where I got it. . . . That was on a Saturday, and I went and saw him on a Monday. I told him and he told me that he had just tested positive three weeks before and he didn't know how to tell me. He thought he got it from me. So it is not that we blamed each other, but neither one of us knew where we had gotten it, which was really weird to me. And I think the relationship was in its final stages. . . . A couple of months after that. . . right after I got sober, his sponsor in AA who is also HIV positive. He said, "My sponsor is HIV positive, and he is someone you can talk to, to be educated and find support." His sponsor said, "Well you know, Brett has been positive since February." "What do you mean?" That's when it all came out, and that's when Brett slipped and said, "I thought I told you that." At that time there was no going back, and Brett couldn't get out of it then. And so, that was the end of the relationship.

Josh tried to establish other sexual relationships. He wanted to make friends with others his age who were also living with HIV. He avoided HIV-related activities because most of the people participating in groups were older.

I don't really like them, because they are generally older people, and I have enough older friends. I would like to make some friends my own age, but people my age really just don't come out and make themselves known. Although I am getting older, you know. When I was twenty-one, twenty-two, twenty-three, you just didn't see people my age in those meetings. There would be twenty-five or thirty people, and there would be one or two my age.

Josh recognized his own social invisibility and the accompanying denial that he and other youths living with HIV and AIDS who were "alone together" experienced.

I think they are withdrawn. There is still a stigma attached to being HIV positive and being young. I think a lot of them are still in the bars and doing different things because they do not see the importance of support groups. . . . There is a lot of denial. Twenty-three, twenty-four, you would rather go out dancing than to a support group.

By late 1994, Josh had not engaged in sexual activity for more than a year; however, he said, "I am sure that I could go out and get laid." He rarely dated, and he avoided gay bars, clubs, or other meeting places. Given his past experiences, truthfulness and honesty were important characteristics of a potential relationship.

I have dated people within this last year and a half, but it just never got to a sexual point for me. I am looking for someone with whom I could be compatible and all that stuff. Companionship. I am not looking for a sexual partner. That's a plus, but I am *looking for a friend*. I want a relationship where both people are honest and respect one another and have compassion for one another, and really just get along. Appreciate one another, learn from each other, grow with someone.

Josh continued to attend AA meetings on a regular basis in the suburbs and worked three jobs to pay his rent and junior college tuition. None of these jobs were related to HIV or AIDS. The job he enjoyed most was working with children at a day care center. Although he liked his privacy, like others, he felt personally responsible for AIDS prevention and education. For example, he was featured in a broadcasted report on HIV and AIDS. He recreated his disclosure to his parents, family, and friends. In hindsight, he had not anticipated the consequences the broadcast would have. He thought that his coming forth and disclosing his status would in some way help other people. However, according to Josh, he was portrayed "irresponsibly" in the program when the producers only used two minutes to represent his life and eliminated all explanatory information about why his life had evolved the way it had. As a result of the broadcast, he lost his anonymity and control over his privacy. People he had casual but ongoing contact with, who did not know of his HIV status before, as a result of the broadcast, knew more about him than he had wanted. His parents had moved a few months earlier, and were unaware of his HIV infection until the broadcast made it necessary for Josh to tell them. He had kept this secret for over a year and a half while he was living at home. He told them over the telephone the week before the broadcast. His family's response to his infection was supportive; his mother was especially concerned and protective.

> I think she thinks I'm dying, and my dad's been a positive person, kind of a strong person. He's like, you know, "You can fight this thing; you can beat this thing." That's kind of my attitude. And my sisters and my brothers–I haven't talked about it with them at that much length, but I think they all pretty much feel the same way. I think my mom, just because she is my mother, tends to look at the downside of it.

Some of his friends knew of his HIV status before, others did not. Most eventually found out.

> Some do; some don't. It depends on when I first found out. I didn't tell them, my friends. I only told my one good friend. I told another really good friend, but I told him not to tell any-one. But it turned out that it really had upset him, and he told his lover. And then he told another friend and my group of friends–not all of them–but they pretty much had the idea, just because all my drinking and how my lifestyle changed. I was really withdrawn for awhile, and they had the idea that I was positive. So when I finally came out and told them, which was

almost a year after I had found out, they knew–some of them knew.

The broadcast also affected his job at the day care center, as he described in detail.

We had a couple of parents withdraw their kids from day care. Some negative letters were written. . . . The district had a letter prepared from the principal of my school to be sent to all of the parents at my elementary school. I said that they should send the letter out before the show aired, and they chose not to. They waited and they let the show go on the air to see who saw it. I didn't like the way they chose to do it. I can't blame them. They didn't know how to handle the situation. It turned out to be trouble because the next day there were a couple of kids who had even seen it, and they asked, "Josh do you have AIDS?" And they were like, messy. So the principal ordered all the children to be told that day–let's get this out. And they sent that letter that day. Well, what happened then was that all these kids went home, and their parents asked, "How was your day?" "Oh fine; Josh is HIV positive." And the parents asked "Who is that?" The parents who knew me were like, "What?" They weren't prepared for their kindergartners coming home telling them about HIV. . . . After everything aired, most people came up to me, and I had parents write letters to the office stating, "I don't know how this is going to go, but I want to go on record that I support Josh."

Josh described the children's reaction and his response.

I'd be asked, "Do you have AIDS?" I said, "No, there is a difference; I am HIV positive." Then I tell them what AIDS is–I just give them a quick spiel. Most of them understand that, and grasp that–it's funny, even a young kindergartner. "I know you just have the HIV; you're okay." I mean, it's nice. It is a tearjerker with some of those kids. Some of the kids were crying and we had a big meeting at day care. My boss said, "You talk to the kids yourself because they have all been told by their teachers, and I can't have kids coming up to me. Let's have a period where you talk to the kids." I talked to them briefly, then they gave me their comments. Some of the younger ones were overwhelmed. We have one little boy who is really intelligent. He says "I know this HIV thing can lead to death, and I don't want you to die." A six-year-old is saying that, and my boss is starting to cry. She said, "That's enough; we don't want everyone crying." A couple of the younger boys that I am close to just live with their moms. I have a lot that are really close to me. One boy got hysterical and they had to take him to the office, and he had a really hard time adjusting to it. His mom talked to him a lot and I talked to him a lot. . . . They still ask me how I got it, and I can't really say that stuff to children. I just tell them, "How I got it is not important. What is important is that I am doing okay now." They asked me how they could get it, and I said they didn't want anyone else's blood getting in contact with them. That is pretty much how you leave it at the elementary level.

Even though Josh was public about his HIV infection, he did not allow his life to evolve around his HIV status. He confronted HIV-related problems only as they occurred, and was resigned to what the future held. In 1994, his T-cell count stood at 700 and suddenly began to drop. His physician suggested that he take AZT. As Josh explained, he was against taking AZT: "I don't want to take AZT now. I don't look at it as an aid; I look at it as the enemy." The change in his T-cell count brought HIV and AIDS into the forefront of his thoughts, and made him confront issues he had thus far avoided.

I've been HIV positive and asymptomatic–not that I've been in denial, but the reality hasn't really set in. I guess now looking back, I thought I had dealt with it. Obviously, this is another reality check. This disease is real. It's like, okay, you're HIV positive for three and a half years. I'm asymptomatic; my count's high; yeah, I'm HIV positive–what does that mean? Nothing really–it doesn't really mean anything to me. And then all of a sudden my count is down, and my physician wants me to start taking AZT. It's like HIV is right in my face. It's like you are sick; that's what it is to me. You have this disease; you are dying. I mean those were the first things that went through my head, and then I got angry. I was a little sad. It was like I was positive all over again. Because you get to a stage where you are real comfortable–or I had gotten–and you just don't expect the count to go down. I thought, "I'll never take medication," and then the doctor suggested that, and it was a big shock. It's only been three and a half years. There have been people who've been asymptomatic going on nine or ten years.

Exercising choice and maintaining control, Josh opted for natural treatments. He took megadoses of vitamins, beta carotene, and anti-oxidants, and exercised at a gym on a regular basis. He saw a physician every four months at the county clinic. After his parents relocated, he moved in with two heterosexual women who knew that he was gay, but did not know that he was living with HIV. Living in the suburbs, he was able to maintain an identity separate from his HIV status and had more occupational and social role options. He was stable, self-supportive, and chose the anonymity and role diversity available in the suburbs. He had future plans that included finishing college and becoming a professional writer. He enjoyed going to museums and reading Greek mythology. Being gay and without a partner in the suburbs was difficult for Josh. He had few opportunities to meet other young people with similar preferences. Maintaining sobriety for Josh also meant avoiding social settings where alcohol was used.

It's like a double-edged sword. I don't go out, because you don't meet very interesting people in the bars. But then I never meet people, so I stay home a lot. I don't know what to do. The gay lifestyle kind of sucks that way. Because when you're straight, you can meet someone at the market or at the work-place. People are so obviously openly straight. We live in a straight society. Everywhere you go, you're going to run into potential people. . . . Gay people are just so closeted. I'm closeted. I mean, I'm not walking around and people think, "Oh, he's gay." The opportunities are a lot less. Your chances are a lot smaller. A lot of people look at the bars as a way to meet people. That is one of the ways to meet people, but not quality people.

More transient youths living with HIV are less interested in, or committed to, suburban life and seek the services more easily available in AIDS magnet urban centers. Others come from financially stable suburban families to which they remain financially and emotionally dependent. As in Josh's case, the financial and sometimes social benefits and advantages of living with or near family members are many. However, the corresponding emotional and psychological costs and disadvantages through masking of self-identity and loss of privacy are equally problematic. These issues for Josh were similar to those from David's recollections.

Chapter 5

"Making Up for Lost Time": David

Why should I seek to ease intense desire
With still more tears and windy words of grief,
When heaven, or late or soon, sends no relief
To souls whom love hath robed around with fire?

Why need my aching heart to death aspire,
When all must die? Nay, beyond belief
Unto these eyes would be both sweet and brief,
Since in my sum of woes all joys expire!

Therefore because I cannot shun the blow
I rather seek, say who must rule my breast,
Gliding between her gladness and her woe?

If only chains and bands can make me blest,
No marvel if alone and bare I go
An armed Knight's captive and slave confessed.

—Michael Angelo Buonarroti, *Love's Lordship* (In Symonds, 1878)

David was an intelligent, twenty-five-year-old gay white male, born and raised in an upper-middle-class, Protestant, West Coast family. His father was a physician and his mother a homemaker. He was among the top students of his high school class. He recalled that there was no STD or AIDS education in the curriculum at his high school.

> When I was in high school, this was earlier in the epidemic and everything, we really didn't discuss AIDS in high school specifically. What I heard was on television, and it was something that happened to these forty-year-old men who lived in San Francisco.

31

David was well dressed and intentionally maintained a "preppie" appearance. He was well traveled, having lived for months in Europe and the Middle East. He reported having used marijuana and snorting cocaine in high school, and described his high school years as a "feisty little horny period" when he was a "man-boy." The first times he had sex with a male and later a female, he "dropped acid." He smoked cigarettes and enjoyed alcohol on a regular basis. His first sexual experiences occurred at age seventeen.

> I hadn't been with another male until I was seventeen years old, and it was simply the fact that I had seen this guy and had an open sexual relationship with him. We had unsafe sex–if you want to think of it in that way–and I knew it.

Asked to elaborate on what he meant by "an open sexual relationship," he explained:

> We were sexually open with each other; we didn't hold anything back, so whatever there was to do in a homosexual relationship, we did. Which of course would have put me in a situation where, you know, I could have gotten HIV positive, that type of thing. So I went and I got tested.

Their openness did not include discussions of STDs, AIDS, or safer sex.

> Well, I was the recipient, and we had anal sex. Essentially I never did it to him; he did it to me. And that had never happened before. As a boy essentially, which is what I was emotionally, I thought I was making him happy.

David discovered that his partner was having sex with other seventeen-year-olds. This "betrayal" forced David to end the relationship. He was tested for HIV soon after, and the test results were negative. He had no further contact with that partner, and eventually he reevaluated the relationship.

> He was twenty-seven. I look back at it now and I really feel taken advantage of. I mean, I was really honestly a naive kid

from the suburbs. I was an intelligent kid and everything else, but at seventeen, I didn't really know what I was doing. A twenty-seven-year-old man saw a cute, little seventeen-year-old, and he had a good time. I can see all of that now.

David amended his use of the term "relationship." "You couldn't call it a relationship, it wasn't mature enough." He also had his first sexual experience with a woman soon thereafter.

She thought it was funny. She was older than I was. In fact, she's probably about thirty now, I would imagine. She was like a friend, and it was the typical drinking-party type atmosphere and all that. We'd all been laughing and joking around, and I told her before that I'd honestly never had intercourse and all that. Well she thought that was real funny. I mean, she said, "Well, I'm going to show you how this works." . . . So she did and we did, and that was that. I've had sex with a couple of other women since. That was all part of going through college. You have to understand that I was right in the middle of trying to figure myself out–through the whole thing, I was living a double life completely.

He denied his homosexuality, and his denial was also reflected in his attitude toward AIDS.

I think I really honestly thought that being gay wasn't necessarily going to be my destiny. It wasn't necessarily where I'd end up. It just seemed like something I would do. I had the same attitude about AIDS that I had about the homosexual acts that I'd participated in, which was, that it wasn't real to me.

His attitude changed as he had more homosexual encounters in college.

I never took AIDS seriously, never even thought about it. But then as I began to get involved and meet more people in the gay community I decided, "Oh well, the thing to do is get tested." . . . As soon as I was around the gay community, I started to be exposed to people handing out condoms in front of bars, to people talking about it, and so it was coming more to the forefront of my mind.

He subsequently moved to the Northwest, transferred colleges, and continued his education. He chose the Northwest because he had friends already living there, and he knew there was a large, accessible gay community.

> I just partied and had a good time. Of course, at that time, I wasn't HIV positive. . . . I was just having a great old time. I wasn't thinking about what I was doing.

David continued to have unprotected sex with men but never discussed AIDS or precautions with his sexual partners. He tried to "play it safe" by selecting partners who fit a certain social profile.

> More conservative than your average gay person. Like I always looked for another young preppie. In my mind, that was somehow safer or something. I mean, it's amazing the games we play with ourselves as human beings.

Short of money and wanting to escape a bad relationship with a short-term lover, David returned south to attend a small, conservative college. He tested again at age twenty-one. Again, he tested negative.

> You'd think that after I had tested negative twice and all that, that I would have had the good smarts to—whatever. That's not the way it worked out. So unfortunately, I learned the reality of everything too late, at least in terms of getting infected. The positive side being that I've learned on the second half of this journey, now that I'm infected . . . everything with regards to what I have to do now, ahead of time. I think I'm *making up for lost time.*

David missed the excitement of the life he had led in the Northwest, and returned there. He began studies in a private law school, and quickly "plugged into" the more affluent, nearby gay community.

I'd drive down to the gay bars and hang out there. It always seems to work out this way for me. I started to get to know all of these older gay men who lived in Lakeview and then people my own age because of my family connections and educational background. I didn't have a hard time getting in with the more well-to-do crowd there within the gay community. And so the next thing I know, I was going to gay parties. . . . People were interconnected.

While continuing his law studies, partying, and engaging in homosexual encounters, David began to meet more "affluent, attractive" people who were living with HIV or AIDS, and he started thinking more about HIV and AIDS.

All these things started plugging into my head. I stayed home from school one day cause I wasn't feeling well, and I watched this HBO [Home Box Office] special. And, not feeling well that day, and putting everything together, I thought, "Gee, I should go get tested because I don't even know what I'm doing." I would go out and look at all these people who are HIV positive. They're attractive and rich, which means it can happen to anybody; you know what I mean?

David was in a new relationship and had a lover when he decided to get tested for a third time at the county health department. His subsequent experiences are quoted in detail.

It was totally different from the first two times I got tested. I knew, somehow. I knew I had had unsafe sex the last two times before I had gotten tested. But you know how we have almost that Jungian sixth sense–it's so strange–as we are as human beings? It was a totally different experience, and when I went back two weeks later, I was just shaking. I'll never forget this moment in my life. This is so ingrained in my head. I remember looking down the hallway at this lady coming with a clipboard, and thinking to myself, "I am not going to walk out of this hospital the same. I know she's going to tell me I'm positive." It wasn't, like, "Oh, I just know I'm positive." It was just knowing. And I went in there and she told me I was. I said,

"I know," and I burst into tears. . . . She left me so helpless by her lack of education and everything else. . . . There's a lot of people she might have sat down and told how much hope there is and everything else. . . . With my education, the way my personality is, I would have listened to her. But she didn't tell me any of the facts.

Following notification, David stopped going to classes, quit law school, avoided his lover, and started drinking, "just vegging out under a twelve pack." In his words, he ended the only "true" relationship he had ever had without explanation. He moved back home to his parents to save money and get his "head together." He told his parents he had been "partying too much," and was "spiritually confused." According to David, his self-concept took a "dive."

At the point that I found out I was HIV positive, first of all, I thought no one would ever want to touch me again. I mean that was one of my initial responses. I also knew that I could never live with myself—I couldn't just go out there and act like everything's normal and start going to bed with people. I knew that even if I ever did have a relationship again someday, it would have to be after I told someone that I was HIV positive. That was so unthinkable, because I felt like such a leper. . . . I had no desire for sex for a number of months there, well actually the physical desire. I was just sick about the whole thing. I just didn't even want it. . . . I was so heavily emotionally affected.

Back in the suburban Southwest, David contacted former college professors and applied and was accepted back into his former college in a Master's degree program. He wanted to get more information about AIDS, and he took precautions so his parents would not discover his HIV status.

I got a post office box so that things wouldn't come to my parents house. And all this information—I started reading all these things. I'm thinking, okay, I need to find out what my T cells were. Because all I knew at that point was that I was HIV-positive. I needed to find out what my T cells were.

David contacted all of the AIDS organizations starting with the National Centers for Disease Control Hotline, which referred him to local AIDS organizations. Eventually he went to see a counselor at a small community-based AIDS services project.

> That day I met Jane. She gave me a hug, and I didn't even know her. I told her I was frightened and I didn't know what to do, but that I had read things, and I felt like I had to do something. I said that I want to go on with my life, and it all started there, and she told me where to go for support groups. She was just there for me. I mean she took a personal interest in what was going on, pointed me in the right directions. Every time I go there, she hugs—she just doesn't sit in her office, she stands in the hallway as if she doesn't have a million things to do. . . . She'd stand in the hallways and then she'd see me and she would remember my name—I couldn't believe that.

With the financial support of his parents, David lived alone in an expensive apartment in an affluent beach community. He rode his bicycle and wrote poetry daily. He received health services from "a state-of-the-art, comprehensive treatment and clinical research center" specializing in early intervention and providing medical treatment, clinical trials, and psychological and nutritional services. Their organizational philosophy coincided with his own. He was determined to take a proactive approach to life with HIV.

> I think we all have our complexes and our little things, and we live in this wonderful dysfunctional society. I think that when you take seriously how finite life is, you start saying, "Wait a minute, I don't want to waste my time here." I don't have another ten years to work through my adolescence. . . . I mean, in a general sense, we all want to be happy and everything. I think I'm more realistic in my expectations about what I expect out of life. I think that the successful life at this point would be to just enjoy each day, and get up and take on new projects, and make the most of the process. I think I've begun to look at life as a process. You never get to wherever it is you're going. Life is what we do every day. So I think enjoying it and making that worthwhile is kind of my general goal now.

Because, before, I was always working toward something. Life was where I was going to get to. Whereas, suddenly I realized how finite life is; life is now and I've got to enjoy it now.

David, in coming to terms with his own life and future activities, was critical of some of the other gay men he saw at the health clinic and differentiated his behaviors from theirs.

I've seen people at the clinic, and then saw them, like, at a bar, just hanging off of five people's necks or whatever. . . . I mean, I have friends. You know, I have some friends that I know at these bars. In the gay community–I'll run up and hug them, give them a big kiss on the cheek in a very platonic way. . . . It's one thing to pal around with friends and put your arms around somebody, give them a big hug. Then there are people who go around bar-slutting, and you know the difference and what's going on. I sometimes think, "Oh my gosh, I saw that guy at the clinic; what's he doing?"

David reentered law school and expected to graduate within a year. He was a member of a Gay Young Republicans Club. Since his family was upper middle class, he was conscious of his position of relative privilege and the accompanying responsibilities. That self-consciousness and his realization of the plight of others contributed to his new identity.

Since this has happened to me, there are so many different people who are dealing with this disease, some of the new friends that I've met have augmented my old friends. I have seen people from different backgrounds with different needs. I think for me as a gay male, I never came out even to myself, really, as gay until this disease shocked me into realizing who I was. I really had a lot in common with a lot of people that I didn't think or didn't want to think I had things in common with.

Altruistic activities represented an important outlet for David to psychologically cope with his HIV status. He had not discussed his homosexuality or HIV status with either of his parents, but believed that "they knew" because of his many AIDS-related volunteer activities. He redefined his career goals from business and making money to helping people living with HIV or AIDS. He spent much of his free time in AIDS work. He volunteered with community-based AIDS organizations delivering food to homebound AIDS patients and working in a legal clinic to promote the rights of those diagnosed with HIV and AIDS. Through these experiences, he knew of the increasing need for AIDS-related education and prevention in suburban areas.

> It needs to happen not just in urban areas; it needs to happen everywhere. And that might take prying a few conservative PTA members out of their seats in suburbia, but I think that even those conservative PTA members are beginning to be realistic about what's going on. Things are different now because it's really affecting everyone's life more. More and more people now know somebody either directly or indirectly who are HIV positive or have AIDS. Living here, dealing with people on a day-to-day basis, people talk about it all the time and not as something that goes on only in large cities. Where I lived, I was completely mentally sheltered and never thought it could happen to me. No one was really telling me that it really could happen to me . . . in a way that was real to me.

Even though David kept very active, he believed that HIV "can be a very lonely disease even if you're surrounded by friends–it's still a very isolating, emotionally isolating thing." Most of his college friends did not know that he was gay. Many close friends who knew that he was gay did not know he was living with HIV. He made new friends through his involvement in AIDS volunteer work or participation in HIV-peer support programs. He dated a few men after his diagnosis, all of whom had tested HIV positive. David wanted a relationship but did not take actions necessary to realize one.

> There are personal issues and little nuances of understanding that I would appreciate giving to and receiving from somebody else who was HIV positive. . . . I would have to work hard to have any kind of sex life with somebody who was HIV negative because of the constant concern that I would have that something would go wrong, and that individual would become

infected and would blame me or something? Whereas, with somebody who's HIV positive, it's just as important to have safe sex because being reinfected is dangerous. But I think it would be wonderful to date someone. We now have seminars where they actually talk about things you can do as a sero-mixed couple. . . . what you can do to be able to be intimate and share with each other.

Despite his lack of a lover or sexual partner, David led an active life and had plans for the future. He emphasized "I don't have time to have AIDS." He was not fully comfortable with his homosexuality. Nevertheless, he was increasingly moving out of the suburban closet. Through AIDS activism and volunteerism, his social network had grown. He intellectualized his worries and fears about his condition, without addressing these concerns directly. The benefits of life in the suburbs for David were his close proximity to his family and their ongoing financial support. In addition, he had friends there that he had known his entire life, and the environment was familiar and safe. Paradoxically, his family and friends were unaware of significant aspects of his life: his homosexuality and his HIV status. His gay friends knew he was homosexual, but most were unaware that he was living with HIV. He led a multifaceted but compartmentalized life, as student, friend, son, homosexual, and young adult living with HIV. The social roles David played were diverse and complex. Yet, the psychological and existential costs to David in having to manage the multiple and often separate and accompanying role identities were high, for even when he was among family and friends, he frequently felt lonely and alone.

Josh and David typify male homosexuals living with HIV and AIDS in the suburbs. In the following chapter, Marie's recollections illustrate the particular and complex struggles that young heterosexual women living with HIV and AIDS experience. Gender-based differences on appropriate sexual behaviors and sexuality exist. Deception, manipulation, and other power imbalances characterized most sexual relationships that the young women studied engaged in, whether in urban or suburban settings. Compared to Josh and David, Marie's experiences highlight the realities facing heterosexual women living with HIV and AIDS.

Chapter 6

"The Courage to Heal": Marie

*If some one has suffered, I feel it not. If some
one has loved, I love more. I sing of my flesh
and my life, and not of the sterile shadow of
buried loves.*

*Remain couched, O my body, according to
your voluptuous mission. Delight in your
daily pleasure and in your passions without
tomorrow. Leave not a joy untasted, to regret
it on the day of your death.*

—Bilitis, *I Sing of My Flesh and My Life* (In Louys, 1920)

Marie was an energetic, twenty-two-year-old white heterosexual female born on the West Coast. She was a veteran of years of psychotherapy and counseling and often spoke in the therapeutic vernacular. In her own words, she came from a "very dysfunctional, complicated family." Marie's parents divorced when she was eighteen months old. Her biological father was a church elder. She had no contact with her biological father during her early childhood. After her parents' divorce, her mother remarried. Her stepfather was mentally, physically, and sexually abusive.

My stepfather abused me when I was three until I was, like, four. I guess I told my mom, and she confronted him, and he denied it and said it was a neighbor. She didn't believe me; she believed him. So I told her that Daddy had a pee-pee thing, or no, I told her that he makes me squeeze and pull his, you know. . . I blocked that out of my memory until she left him for the first time—she left four different times. The first time she left him we were driving to my grandparents' house and all of a sudden the memory clicked–I just remembered it and it was like it happened yesterday. It was like I hadn't remembered it for a long time. I told my mom, and she said, "I'm never going back together with him." Then later on, again, she confronted him. He denied it and then we went to counseling, and the counselor told me that I was fantasizing, that I made it up. The counselor told me that.

Marie was consistently abused throughout her childhood and early adolescence. Conflicts often arose out of normal daily activities, such as when she would exert independence by refusing to eat.

I would never swallow my food. I just wouldn't want to swallow it. I'd sit there for an hour with my cheeks puffed out like a chipmunk with all this food. I would cry, and I would get into big trouble. I'd go and throw up and I'd get in trouble for throwing up. My mother would just stand there, and she wouldn't protect me or anything–it was really awful. I used to be really, really, really skinny. . . . But it was awful, and he [her stepfather] would degrade me at the table. At the table when we were eating, we'd always get into fights because I always would stick up for myself instead of just being quiet–fight back–and get in more and more trouble. He would end up saying, "You're nothing but a fourteen-year-old, duh duh duh, leave the table." And so I'd go off crying. He was a real jerk.

Marie had a stepbrother and a stepsister. Both, she believed, were similarly abused.

Well, it was awful. They went through hell, too. My brother would try to hold my mom's hand and my dad would knock the hand out. He was really abusive to my brother too, probably sexually. There are just some things that I see in my brother, and I go, "Oh, that's kind of strange." So he was probably sexually abused too. I know for sure that my sister was. She never told me, but when she was little, old enough to change her clothes, she would change her clothes constantly. I know little kids do that, but she would wear five and six pairs of underwear at the same time, and she would constantly change them.

At age fourteen, Marie ingested a large quantity of aspirins and went to school. She laughed in recalling that at that time, she thought "you could kill yourself with aspirins." She also started to have sex at age fourteen. Her first sexual experience as she recalls, was not pleasurable.

> It was awful. . . . All my friends were having sex and I felt left out–not all of my friends, but a lot of my friends that I hung out with. So one day I was coming home from school and this one guy that I liked a lot, he said, "Come over to my house," I didn't know what to do. He gave me a brandy, and then we like. . . It wasn't even special, I felt I was being raped or something. I didn't like it. Then I had sex with him again and with his friend. . . . He wanted to have a three-way with me, him, and his friend. . . . I didn't know what that was, I didn't know what to do. . . because I had been sexually abused when I was little. I didn't know that I could say no, or that I had a right to my own body or anything. I didn't want to do it, but I did it just because I don't know. I couldn't say no. I didn't know that I could say no. It was awful, it was just awful. . . . There was no foreplay; they just got on top of me and did it. I just laid there.

Marie had adjustment problems in school even though she made many friends. Her mother finally divorced her stepfather when Marie was fourteen, which she remembers as a significant event. She remained angry at her mother for failing to protect her from her stepfather.

> She knows that it's true. The abuse was true, but she says, "Oh, he didn't really mean to do it, he was abused as a kid, too. He just did the things that were done to him, to you. He really loved you." She minimizes it all. . . . She didn't believe that it happened until the last few years. It's because she didn't want to own the fact that I was being abused and that she didn't take care of me and wasn't protecting me. She also was abused when she was a kid. I didn't find that out until recently. . . . She

doesn't deal with it, so she's pushing it down, pretending it's not true. And I hate how she raises my brother and my sister. She always made me take care of her. She made me the mom. . . . She would tell me that my stepfather was stealing. She would tell me things about my stepfather, and then I would have to live with him, knowing these things. She would ask me for advice: "What do you think I should do? Do you think I should leave him?. . . Okay, I'm going to leave him." And then she'd go back on her word. She would ask my advice and then she wouldn't take it. I'd get really angry. Then when she divorced him and she had another boyfriend and she was living with him and I was living with her and him, she would tell me about their sex life and their problems, and what a jerk he was. I had to live with him, and I used to like him. Now, I'm sitting there hating him and thinking he's a jerk but trying to get along with him, too. It ruined our relationship. She was never there for me emotionally. I was always there for her. If I was upset or crying, I would call her and we would talk for five minutes and then for half an hour we would talk about her. I just couldn't deal with it anymore. I tried to get rid of all the toxic people in my life. She was the most toxic!. . . I always try to fix people, and I tried to fix her. All my life I've been trying to fix her, and I get into relationships–I just got out of a relationship where I was trying to fix her [her mother], and I wanted people to fix me.

Marie graduated from high school and spent two years in college. She stopped speaking to her mother. She recalled in detail particularly hurtful actions of her mother, including one year when she returned home for the holidays.

Right before Christmas, she had my high school graduation picture on the wall. She took that down and she replaced it with pictures of my brother and sister when they were little kids. I saw it because I came and took my sister out for Christmas Eve. I saw my picture was gone and pictures of my sister and brother when they were little were up there. It was like she was eliminating me, like she never had me.

Marie's problems escalated, and she started to drink alcohol more frequently. Shortly thereafter, she went to school intoxicated and was raped. A concerned psychology teacher referred her to a male psychotherapist. She disliked the male therapist, and within a year found a female counselor she preferred. At the time of these counseling sessions, she was in her late teens. She was provided with HIV prevention information.

> The reason I went and saw her was because I was having sex with these guys and I didn't want to. I didn't know how to stop, and I was smoking and I wanted to quit smoking. . . . I was having sex after sex after sex with different guys. . . . It was my escape. I guess you'd say I was a sex addict. That's all because of the abuse when I was little. I went to her to ask her to fix me! "I'm having sex with all these people, and I don't want to. I'm smoking and I want to stop." She helped me to stop smoking and I started again. She made me do all these things. I only had ten weeks with her and she had me do all these things. She had me buy this book, *The Courage to Heal.* She had me get on the waiting list for the women's support group. She had me keep a journal and read all this stuff and she had me listen to this tape. She told me she didn't want me to become HIV positive. So I listened to this tape about how to be assertive and say, "Yes, you should wear a condom."

Marie tested HIV positive in 1990 on her first test. Her counselor encouraged her not to tell anyone "because once you tell someone, you don't know what the reaction will be." Initially, Marie thought this was good advice. At the time of the interviews (three years later), she still carried the printout of her test and HIV-positive results.

> It's kind of ironic, before I was infected, I had a boyfriend who was a virgin and wanted me to get tested before we had sex. I couldn't believe he wanted me to get tested. I wish I would have got tested then—it probably would have made me realize how serious it was. Maybe not—because I was acting out sexually. . . . He wanted me to get tested, and I didn't get tested, and then we had sex. Then I broke up with him because

he drove me crazy. He always wanted to be with me, very controlling and stuff. After that, I met this guy named Giovanni. I was working at The Diner. I just got off work and I met this guy, really good-looking. I was all "Whoa." . . . I ended up staying the night with him. I was a fundamentalist Christian at the time, and I ended up staying the night at his hotel. I offered that he could stay with me because he was running out of money. We didn't have sex that night, but we did kiss. Over a period of three weeks, I fell in love with him, I guess. I don't know if it was real love. He had to go back to Italy to serve his military service because everyone in Italy has to do one year of military service. So, he went back to Italy and then he came back one year later. . . . While he was gone—that's when I started sleeping with all these guys. He lived with me for ten months when I was living with my grandma.

Over time, Giovanni made a number of trips between the United States and Italy, and they maintained a long-distance relationship. Eventually, Giovanni went to the South Pacific to look for work. He would call Marie from there to ask about her "weird" swollen lymph nodes and the rash on her face. Manipulation and deception increasingly characterized their relationship.

He asked me, "How are your lymph nodes?" And I said, "Am I going to die or something?" And he said, "Could be." He said he had to fly from New Zealand in two days to tell me something and then go to Rome or fly back to New Zealand. He didn't know which, and I thought, "Great, he has AIDS!" That's what I thought. And when he came back, he told me that he got a vaccination for hepatitis and before they gave him the vaccination for hepatitis, they tested him—his red-cell count— and . . . it was really low. Then he was tested for AIDS and it came out negative. He wanted to know if I had it because if I had it, it meant that he had it. I'm thinking, "Oh, great!" And so I was kind of worried, and later when he was back, and I was driving to the clinic—we would always fight. I said, "Why don't you get tested, too?" He said "No, I'm not getting tested. You know how much I hate needles." . . . But I wanted him to get tested again. He said "No, I don't want to get tested." I said, "Why not?" because I didn't believe him. I was thinking he came out positive and wants me to get tested now. So, he said, "Take me home; I want to pack my bags and go back to Rome." I said, "Okay, fine." I drove home, dropped him off, and I went and got tested by myself. Two weeks later, we were in another fight, and he was out surfing with his friend. I went and got the results by myself. . . . I came out positive. I still thought he gave it to me. . . . All of a sudden, I was just crying and crying and crying, and he's said, "What's wrong?" And I thought, "Oh my God, I've killed him; he didn't have it." And then I told him I was positive. He started crying, and he cried and cried. He cried more than I did, and I was the one who had to take care of him. It sucked, because I was the one who was positive. Then I found out that he was never tested. He had this dream that I had AIDS, and I was going to die, and that he might also have it. So because of this dream and my swollen lymph nodes, he asked his cousin who is a doctor about AIDS and HIV. He wanted me to get tested, and he never got tested, and so he went and got tested.

Giovanni initially tested negative. Their two-year on-again/off-again relationship ended, and he returned to Italy.

Two days later, he went back to Italy. I never wanted to talk to him again. . . . Then all of a sudden, he got swollen lymph nodes. . . . He had converted to being positive; I think it was within six months. Before that we had sex while I was on my period without condoms. He wouldn't use a condom. I said, "Use a condom because I don't want to get pregnant.". . . Sometimes now I miss him, but we had a really dysfunctional relationship—he was a real jerk. But it was a good thing that he had that dream because it's a good thing that I got tested. I would have hated to wake up in a hospital bed and find out I had AIDS. That would be much worse. I would rather know than not know. I think it would suck to give it to someone else, too. I gave it to him. . . . I know I did, because how else would he get it? Because he came out negative and then he converted to positive. I got it from my manager at work.

During the periods when Giovanni traveled, Marie saw other men, including Evan. Evan was the twenty-eight-year-old "really good-looking" manager of The Diner where she worked as a part-time waitress. In hindsight, she believed he infected her. She identified exactly when she thought HIV infection occurred.

> I had a party, and got real drunk. He was real drunk and he ended up staying the night and we had sex. It was like an all-nighter too. He was on cocaine and he couldn't ejaculate, so it was all night long. It was really long, so I'm sure there were plenty of tears in my tissue for me to get it. And it really sucks that I got it from a one-night stand. The reason I know is four weeks later I had my first yeast infection. I knew he had sex with this other girl–she denies it–she had herpes. I thought, "Oh God, I have herpes." I went to the health center.

Marie later remembered that she had sex with Evan on two occasions, not just one. The night she believed she was infected, she had condoms in the dresser drawer next to her bed. He didn't volunteer and she didn't insist that he use them. Eventually, Marie confronted Evan about her HIV infection.

> I went to his house and I told him I was HIV positive, and I said, "I'm not going to try to blame you and say you gave it to me, or I gave it to you–I don't know which, but you need to go get tested." He said, "Oh man, and I was just starting to feel better, too." And I said, "What do you mean?" And he said, "'Well, I've had diarrhea every day for, like, a year now." And he showed me his arm and he had shingles. . . . I told him that he needed to go get tested. I gave him all this information, card, phone number, and everything. Two or three months later I went back to his house to see if he got tested. I was dying to know. . . . I went to his house and I opened the door and he's in bed with this girl.

Subsequently, Marie got to know this other young woman well. She also was a waitress and later would attend HIV-support groups. Marie believed that like herself, this woman also had been infected by Evan. He had not been forthcoming with either about his HIV status. Marie was angry with Evan and claimed that he had constantly sexually harassed her.

> When I was at work he would always try to get me to sleep with him again. I wouldn't. He would put me in really bad stations. I wouldn't flirt with him or sleep with him. Not because I wouldn't, but when I wouldn't he would be mean to me. But when I did, when I would flirt with him back, he would be nice to me. Then he had this thing, "I have this new idea to reduce stress. The butt is the biggest muscle in the body—so I will massage your butt." He would do that, grab my butt. . . . He did that to several of the waitresses and it really upset me because I couldn't say, "You better not do that." I would have reported him, but I couldn't because I was afraid I'd lose my job. . . . I almost wish I could sue the company for sexual harassment. I don't know if I have a case because they could always say, "Oh well, you slept with him." And they would probably bring up everybody else who I've slept with in my life. There are a lot. Not as many as some of my friends who are negative. I don't know if I could win. Plus, I don't want to bite the hand that feeds me. But by them making me keep it a secret, I feel very angry. I feel that if I had never worked for The Diner, I wouldn't be HIV positive.

One of the biggest challenges for Marie was how to manage her reputation at the franchise restaurant where she worked. Marie had started to go to women's and AIDS support groups and was coming to terms with her health condition. She had spoken publicly about her infection. The reactions she received at work varied but were generally supportive.

> Everyone was supportive. One of my managers cried. He wanted to go with me to a support group. He never did. Everyone was very supportive. Then the home base supervisor came to me and I thought I was in big trouble. Because when I was on the radio I said I worked for a restaurant and I named The Diner. They offered me a job in the corporate office, and I thought, "Cool, I don't have to be a waitress." I took it, but there was a condition—that I wouldn't tell anyone at work that I

> was HIV positive. I didn't like the idea. But well, I didn't know these people anyway. But now I know them and I'm pretty close to them and I'm trying to keep a secret, so that's weird. . . . When I got transferred, they hired me with the condition that "You don't tell anyone, not a single person at work, that you're HIV positive." I said "Okay." . . . They offered me the job because they were afraid that it would cause a controversy and people wouldn't come in and stuff.

Informing her family and personal friends about her HIV infection was not easy. In time, she changed jobs and the process began again.

> There was a time when I told just about everybody. Then my whole life changed . . . because everybody at my work knew, and I changed jobs. Now I don't talk to those people I worked with. In fact, my circle of friends has changed. The circle of friends that I usually see don't know.

Her mother tried to be supportive, but their long-standing problems prevented any real reconciliation. Marie had to create her own support. She saw a therapist twice weekly and attended support groups for survivors of abuse another two days per week. She described how and why she engaged her therapist.

> I asked her if she did regressive work and she said, "Yes." I liked that she was going to be my therapist. But she didn't have that much time because of the women's support group. She wanted to charge me ninety-five dollars a session. I'm, like, "Ninety-five dollars!" She knows how broke I am. That really hurt. I felt abandoned. We worked through that. . . . That's why I'm so poor. It's expensive! It's four hundred and eighty dollars a month for my therapy. A lot of people say to me, "Is it worth it?" "Well, it's either that, or I kill myself or end up in a mental hospital; which do you prefer?" A lot of people don't understand that if I wasn't in therapy, you know, I get suicidal. Like when a new memory is trying to come up or something. I get to this point where I don't want to live—some people get like that. I don't really act on it.

Marie continued to seek, as she said, "good-looking men" with problems, as her most recent love/hate relationship exemplified. Her description of him is telling: "It's not like he's a nice guy who can be a jerk; it's like he's a jerk who can be a nice guy."

> I met this guy who is a hemophiliac and he's HIV positive, and he had a cocaine and an alcohol problem. . . . It's weird, all of the people who come out and say they're HIV positive, we all know each other. He was the best-looking guy at the parties. He was really, really, really good-looking.

Marie met Craig at a party for heterosexuals living with HIV in a suburban town in the Southwest. She was immediately physically attracted to him. Craig was thirty-two and had been a lifeguard for ten years—"Taster's Choice, he's six foot three; he's a babe. The only thing is, he knows it." Craig had recently lost his girlfriend to AIDS, and he was looking to recreate the same relationship with Marie he had experienced with his past lover. In time, Marie and Craig discussed marriage and what it involved if both were living with HIV.

> He wanted me to get pregnant by him and have a baby. I said, "You're crazy." It would make my T cells go down so low. I don't want to die and leave behind a kid. Who is going to take care of this kid? I don't want the same thing to happen to the kid that happened to me." . . . He would say that in five years there's going to be a cure. He might not be around, but I'll be around. . . . He's in so much denial about HIV. . . . I opened up to him more than I opened up to anyone. Like our sex life wasn't that great. He would like to go into the bedroom and then just do it. I would try to tell him, "I need you to touch me this way and touch me like this and like that." He would get all defensive. . . . I had a lot of problems sexually because of the abuse. I had never opened up to a guy that way before.

Marie and Craig had broken up a number of times. Nevertheless, they still went away together on small vacations and occasionally slept together. Finally, Marie decided to put the relationship on "permanent" hold. Marie continued to keep busy, and she was often exhausted by the end of her day. She worked full-time at The Diner's corporate headquarters. She also attended her individual therapy and support groups and baby-sat and painted houses part-time to earn extra money. What little free time she had was spent at the university hospital where she received experimental HIV treatment. She did not respond well to these treatments. She developed severe diarrhea from the didanosine (ddI) she was taking. She was concerned because she had gone off of AZT because of a bad reaction. Her doctors started her on combination AZT and dideoxycytidine (ddC). She lost a lot of weight, her energy level was low, and her overall health declined.

Marie lived in a working class, multiethnic neighborhood a short distance from her grandmother's house, where she did her laundry on a weekly basis. She lived in a one-bedroom apartment with two dogs, two cats, and two goldfish. AIDS-related posters were taped to the walls. She bought a horse, which she housed at a local stable, and rode on weekends. Her pets were an important source of emotional support. She was an organizer of self-help groups for heterosexuals living with HIV. As she was quick to emphasize at the time of the interviews in late 1993, there were very few services that directly targeted heterosexuals living with HIV and AIDS.

> A lot of heterosexuals do not want to go to gay organizations because they are homophobic. So they don't get the support they need. I can relate to that. I want us to be able to offer services to people who are really sick . . . . and who can't go places. Because a lot of people, when they get sick, all their friends stop visiting them. . . . It's too painful. . . . A lot of people stop visiting. So I would like to start an organization, a group of people who would visit people who are sick. It's amazing how many people stop visiting.

At age twenty-two, Marie was successful in starting the group she desired. She concurrently dealt with her own personal adjustment to living with HIV. When she reflected on her past, her self-destructive impulses, including periodic alcohol abuse, resurfaced. Constant activity and activism were methods of controlling her negative impulses. Regardless of her declining condition, she had an astounding amount of vitality at times, both physical and mental, that manifested outwardly in a surprising *joie de vivre*. She had little time or energy or desire to focus on regrets. More significant, through activities, survivors' groups, and individual therapy, she addressed past feelings of inadequacy, powerlessness, childhood experiences of abuse, and an adolescence of casual, oftentimes involuntary sexual activity. In her young adulthood and in how she chose to go about living with HIV, she finally felt more in control. She also faced and responded to blatant institutional discrimination based on gender and HIV status.

> I don't want to hide my things. I don't want to live a life of pretend. That's a big part of my life. It's a very big part of my life. I'm active in talking about it and trying to deal with it and getting information. I don't want to hide everything away, hide part of myself.

Living in the suburbs had both advantages and disadvantages for Marie. Like Josh and David, she was able to blend into the anonymity of suburbia when she wanted. She was forced to hide her health condition from others even though she realized it was an important part of her life. She wanted to be connected to a larger group of young heterosexual people living with HIV and AIDS, but had to travel far to participate in group activities. Her life was particularly complicated as she was a high-profile and public AIDS activist, and well integrated and functioning in more anonymous suburban social and occupational worlds. Her life was very different from Ethan's.

Chapter 7

"That Will Be Extra": Ethan

All but visibly beating
We feel thy wings in the far
Clear waste, and the plumes of them fleeting,
Soft as a swan's plumes are,
And strong as a wild swan's pinions, and swift as the
flash of the flight of a star.

—Algernon Charles Swinburne, *A Dark Month,* 1882

Ethan was an exotic-looking, twenty-three-year-old gay male from a Catholic, Pacific Island family. Tall and stockily built, his crew-cut hair accentuated his facial features. Considered attractive and masculine, Ethan appeared five years older than his actual age. His eyes always appeared gloomy, but he smiled often, displaying crooked, amber-colored teeth stained by years of coffee and cigarette use, and ravaged by the effects of chronic substance abuse. He usually wore colorful and expressive baseball caps or Rastafarian hats. His clothing was a trendy combination of used pieces he had carefully selected at secondhand stores. His jewelry included various oversized finger rings. Around his neck hung multiple chains with skulls and crossbones, large crucifixes with and without Jesus, peace symbols, and ankhs. His speech was rapid, and his thoughts were often disorganized. Most of the time he was either currently running or coming off speed.

Ethan was raised on the West Coast, and his father abandoned his family when he was a young boy. As a child, Ethan was overweight, had brown curly hair, and was considered "an ugly duckling." He would take traditional foods to school for lunch daily. Other children used to ridicule him calling him "fatty" and "green banana eater." He was raised by his mother in a public housing project. His mother was very religious and active in her church (she was one of the "church-going folks"). She remarried but soon separated from Ethan's stepfather. Ethan had a older sister and a younger half-brother. He described his role in the family, which he felt was partly related to his skin color.

> I was more like the soft side. I was the soft side of the family. I would take everything. I would take the beatings. I would take the punishments. I would take the demands, everything that went on in the family, like the stress and the domination. I would be the one responsible for the family's faults. If the family had a problem, it would be either on the adults or on the kids. If it was on the kids, then it was on me. Because of the fact that I was the oldest son in my family, and my brother was the youngest, I had to be a role model for him or something. But the thing was, while I was trying to be a role model for my brother, my sister was my role model. I mean she's bigger than me, and she's taller than me; she's whiter than me.

Ethan knew he was sexually attracted to males from age thirteen. He never had sexual relations with a female. At thirteen, he engaged in sexual activity for the first time with a male, his twenty-seven-year-old uncle.

> It was like when I was thirteen–I was with my uncle. I would do what he wanted me to do. It was weird. This was going on until I was almost fourteen. All of a sudden I caught a liking to it. So all of a sudden it stopped. He didn't want to have sex with me or do anything with me. He would tell me, "Be a man; don't be a girl. Put on some pants and don't wear shorts so much." Every time I would sit there and tell him, "You know it's not my fault. I like to wear what I like to wear, and if I didn't like to wear this, I would wear something different." We would get into arguments, and I would tell him it's because of you that I'm like this. "You're damn lucky your wife doesn't know about this. Because if your wife knows, then she is going to kill you because you have a son." Back

then it was a macho thing. Bully the faggot. Make the faggot do what the straight boy wants to do. It was pathetic.

Ethan kept secret his sexual activity with his uncle. He started running away from home about the same time.

> I ran away. I was having trouble at home, difficulties dealing with the fact that I was gay and my mother couldn't accept that. All these things, growing up and not realizing who my real father was. It was just this one big problem for one kid to deal with and I couldn't deal with it. Going to school and people teasing me because I'm gay. I remember my brother and sister were there. My brother and sister were the only two that would defend me when people called me names. To this day, they are homophobic but not toward me, only toward others.

During his late childhood and early adolescence, Ethan was physically and emotionally abused by his mother. He described her as "really violent." She used "belts, brooms, or anything she could get her hands on" to beat him.

> My mother was very abusive and very demanding. Everything that she wanted done, I would have to do. It was as if anything went wrong with the family she took it out on me. She would do this, and it wasn't my fault. I understood what she was doing; it's my father's fault. That's why I hate him.

Following an occasion when his mother struck him, he was hurt deeply by particularly cruel comments his mother made. He had not forgotten her words or his response in ten years.

> After she was done she said, "Sometimes I wish you were never born. You make me sick. Look at you, you don't even look like a boy. You look like a frickin' girl. Why weren't you born a girl?" Then we went upstairs and went to bed. But I couldn't go to sleep because I was thinking about what she said. I thought to myself, "I can't take this. I'm leaving." So I packed a small duffle bag, two pairs of pants, climbed out of the window, and walked out.

The first time he ran away, he went straight to the area where street-based, commercial, male sex work occurred. He knew where to go because he had been there before.

> Well, I saw it one day when I was taking the bus. I was with my friends. They looked out the window and said, "Look at all these homosexuals and all these faggots. There's a homosexual and he's a prostitute." I thought, "Wow, this is a gay street." I thought maybe I'll come down here some other time. Then that day that my mother beat me up, I just left. I stayed till I was fourteen. . . . She started getting abusive, and I was like, "I can't take this anymore." I told my sister, "I'm leaving." I was running away. My sister said, "Don't run away because you're only going to make things worse. Mom's going to do this, na, na, na, and she's got high blood pressure," and this and that. I said that she shouldn't be beating on me, you know. She knows. "Why is she doing this? Why is she acting like this?" So she was wrong. She hit me, and I left.

Ethan went to the gay area he had seen from the bus, and became a male sex worker at age thirteen.

> I just started walking around. People started giving me money, like two dollars because I was panhandling. Then they said, "Hey, you know you could pull a trick." I'm like, "Whoa, I don't know what that is." I knew what it was. When a person pulls over, and you go with them; you tell them what you want. I was like, "Whoa, okay, I'll do it." That's how I started hustling.

Ethan did not return home, and he stayed for periods of time with the men who picked him up on the street. He met a 48-year-old businessman who supported him for a few months.

> He liked me. He was giving me money, buying me this and that, and I liked it. I told him I didn't want to go back to my family. I felt that I was taking him for what he had. I thought, "I'm going to stay here with this man, and the only reason why I'm doing this is because I want money. Because he buys me things."

While staying at this man's apartment, Ethan still continued his street-based sex work. Various short- and long-term kept situations followed. He met Jordan, an African American, then age fourteen, who became his best friend. Together, with three other youths in a similar situation, they formed a street-based family, as Ethan referred to them, the "crew." All of them were estranged from their families, gay, with impermanent living arrangements, drug dependent, and involved in sex work to pay for their habits. In 1985, Ethan started going to the local social service agency that assisted street youth. The Program was located within a couple of blocks from the area where male sex-workers plied their trade. The Program conducted street-based outreach. At The Program offices, they provided food, short-term housing, and use of a telephone. If his family did not hear from him for a long time, they would contact him through The Program. In a superficial way, Ethan felt connected to the friends he made on the streets. He rarely shared his feelings with them, and considered them "kooks," "leeches," or "space cadets." However, he prefered the closeness of his "crew."

> Wherever there was drugs, wherever there was anything, fun, excitement, and adventure, that's where we would be. There were four of us. There was like a mob of us going around. We were all best friends.

Not long after he used marijuana for the first time, he quickly began using other substances. He started injecting speed, what practitioners on the street call "slamming."

> I was tired of going to sleep and everyone else was walking around and all energetic all night. I asked, "How do you stay up this late?" Jordan says, "Well we just can." Jordan turned me on to it. I snorted first, and I guess I started slamming it later on when I was seventeen or eighteen. I had to get used to how it makes you feel at first, the rush, and everything else. That syrup is slimy. . . . You don't get that intensified rush from snorting that you do from slamming it. But then again, when you slam it, uh, it hurts. Most of the time it hurts.

Ethan would return home after one month on the streets, only to leave again when his mother continued to beat him. He hitchhiked to

Southern California for the first time. He stopped when he saw the Hollywood sign from the freeway. He walked in the direction where he sensed he might find street-based sex work.

> I followed that sign for about two or three hours. It was getting dark, and I was getting hungry. I was cold, and I was tired. So I crashed in a park. I woke up the next morning. I walked and found The Boulevard. There was this guy who was selling drugs. He was selling crack. I asked him, "Do you know where guys go to hustle, to make money?" He said, "That's on The Boulevard. You go down the block." So I walked down there and I found it.

Ethan supported himself as an teenage sex worker in Southern California for the next six months. He started to use crack.

> I was smoking crack. Crack just made me—the dependence you have on that stuff. My eyes were sunken in; I was gross. I didn't look healthy. I was thin and all my clothes didn't fit. I had to give them away. I had to buy new clothes, and they wouldn't fit after I ate. So I gave up crack. I moved back home to my mom. When I got back from Southern California, I stayed with my mom for awhile, three months. I got fat, and back to normal. Then I had enough. I felt the urge to go back out, and party with my friends. It was the weekend. I said "Boy, I'll do it."

Ethan would travel back and forth between Southern and Northern California every three or four months, "I was like a traveling salesman." He would return north to be with his family and friends.

> I would go south and hustle there and make a couple of bucks. I'd stay for God knows how long, until I got tired of it or it got tired of me. Then I would have to leave there and come back here, and do it all over again here. But then I would get burned out here a lot quicker.

When in the North, he would go to The Program for assistance. When in the South, he went to a gay and lesbian service agency. He had to be in "bad shape" in order to seek help.

> I would go there to find a way home, or try to find a place to stay because the streets had really drugged me out. I was so stressed on the streets that I wasn't making any money. I would be staying up all night. I would be sleeping in parks or wherever.

He liked the excitement that went with sex work. In a short period of time, he built up a clientele he would call upon for help, and stay with for periods of time when necessary. When one "gig" would end, he would move on to another. His customers were mostly older men and reflected his preference in sexual partners.

> That started when I came out of the closet I guess. I was more attracted to older men than to younger men. It was a mental thing. Like you know the old saying, the older you get, the wiser you get? I figured if I'm attracted to older men, then they would help me along with life. Because they are wiser about what's going on, what's good and what's bad, what's right and what's wrong. It's like they were teaching me. That's why I like older men. Younger guys are more "Hey, let's party, let's go buy cars, clothes, and spend time at the movies."

Jordan introduced Ethan to his first "real boyfriend" Ray in Northern California. Ethan was fourteen and Ray was twenty-five. There was an immediate attraction. Ray let it be known that he had just broken up with his last boyfriend. Ethan flippantly responded that he would be interested in "applying for the job," depending upon "the size" of Ray's wallet.

> Ray would show up every once in a while, sometimes two or three times a week and come down and see me. He would bring all these new things. Everything he had was brand new, fresh right out of the store. He would have new watches, new clothes, new credit cards, gold cards, and this and that. He would spend most of what he had on me. I thought at the time, having a boyfriend, having an older boyfriend who was richer than I was, was cool. But then a little birdie told my friends, and my friends told me, that this guy was bad news. At the time I didn't believe them. I didn't want to believe them. We

hadn't had sex. We had been going out for about a year, and we didn't have sex. He would give me things, and he would buy me things. He was buying me things and giving me things that were stolen. All the cards, and all these other things he would have, they were stolen. I didn't know it.

Ray became Ethan's episodic boyfriend, and eventually his lover for the next two years. Monogamy or exclusivity were never characteristics of Ethan's relationships. He continued street-based sex work. By 1986, the fear of AIDS had spread faster than HIV infections. The economic opportunities and advantages of street-based sex work declined. Many sex workers were setting up answering services or voice mail, and advertised in gay-oriented newspapers and magazines to identify, attract, and engage customers. Male sex work shifted from the streets to more removed, anonymous, escort or male model services. For Ethan, who did not have stable housing or resources, sex work on the streets remained his only viable option. His competition increased.

At the time, AIDS was already announced, so everybody was really hype. This thing called AIDS, we didn't want to catch it. Nobody wanted to die. There were more hustlers and there were less tricks. Tricks thought, "I'm not going to pick this one because he looks like he has AIDS."

Ethan described a regular customer of his at the time. The protective actions and rescue fantasies of his clients, tricks, or johns contrasted with Ethan's own intentions. The nature of the competition among sex workers was also evident in Ethan's description.

We would meet near City Hall. He would take me to lunch, or he would take me to dinner. Then we would go back to his place. I would do my little business there with him. He hated it like that you know. But he gives me money for sexual favors, and I hate the fact that I have to have sex for money. We sat there one night and we had this big two- or three-hour conversation about why I do it. "I do it because I have to do it. I do it because there is no other way for me. Because if there was, I would do it." So I told this guy that, and he started acting like a protector. He would tell me, "Well, I don't want to see you out there. So if you want to spend the night, whatever. I don't want to see you out on the street. If you need money, I will give you money. When you leave here, maybe you can correct this, and then you can do whatever later". . . . So, should I stay, or should I go? I didn't know what I wanted. I had more problems going on in my life than just having to deal with the streets. . . . I'm sitting here with this guy, I would sleep with this guy, and he would give me eighty bucks. And that was only for what—I would do things for him. I would stay in his house because I didn't want to go out anymore. I had been up for a whole day, or I hadn't slept all night. Or, I just didn't feel like going out anymore. The next morning I would wake up and leave his house. I would go back to the streets and I would run into my friends. I wanted to treat my friends to breakfast. They go, "No, no, no, we'll treat you to breakfast." And it's like, "Well, wait a minute. How long have you been out there?" They say they've been out there all night. They've pulled four or five dates, and they've made this much money. I say, "Why do you do this? I could have made a little bit less or a little bit more, right, with more tricks last night if I didn't spend the night with him." Then that becomes a problem for me. I would turn every little thing into a problem and stress my life, and make my life a lot worse.

In his middle and late teens, Ethan had to earn money daily given his lack of resources and housing. He was a sex worker at all times, and whenever possible, he would make a social situation into a moneymaking opportunity. A day at the beach was a good example. Ethan went to a gay beach with a friend, and left with a twenty-five-year-old blond named Christopher who he lived with for two months.

I met this guy and he's nice. He's blond and had blue eyes. We went back to his place. I told him, "Well, I don't feel comfortable." I thought, "Let me see if I can work this and make this guy give me money, instead of just having sex for free." All I had that day was sixty bucks. I had already blown twenty bucks for bus fare, snacks, cigarettes, and stuff like that on the way to the beach. And forty dollars wasn't going to be enough to pay for rent. When I told this guy that I was a hustler, this guy just freaked, and I asked, "Are you okay?" He asked, "Well, what were you doing at the beach?" I said, "I thought it was a nice day so I decided to take a break." He laughed and thought that was funny. "I didn't want to tell you that I hustle for money. I didn't want to tell you this either, but I'm short on my rent, and I'm also kind of short on money for food and stuff like that." I'm going on and on. He explained why he can't give me money. He only had so much. I said, "Then what's the plan?" I told him since it's not working, I told him I don't feel like having sex. "I mean I do want to have sex, but you know, I'm thinking more of myself, because I need a place to stay, and my rent is due in the morning and I don't have enough." I told this guy that and he said, "Okay, I'll see what I can do." He asked me if I wanted to stay for awhile, or if I wanted to do something. I said, "Well, I don't know. What do you think? Obviously I'm putting you in a very awkward position and I don't normally do that. But, it's best that I tell you the truth now than you find out later." I told him "I'll stay with you. I'll have sex with you. But you have to give me what I need."

He stayed with Christopher that night. Ethan was paid eighty dollars for oral sex, which he spent on rent, food, and drugs. After the first night, he did not charge for sexual favors. He also did not turn down whatever was offered.

All of a sudden I started feeling attached to him because of the way he looked. He was cute. He was single. He liked me. I told him that I liked him, and I shouldn't have done what I did the first time I met him. I didn't want his money. It was more like if he could give me what he could, fine. But only if I ask for it. If I don't ask for it, I don't need it.

Ethan was soon evicted from his hotel, and moved in with Christopher. Christopher bought Ethan new clothing, and took him on long automobile drives. Ethan enjoyed the friendship, but was less enthusiastic about the sex.

I would wake up in the middle of the night handcuffed, with my legs tied to the bedpost with him lying on top of me kissing me and all sorts of things. He would say, "Don't worry, I'll take them off." I didn't know this guy was this much in heat. And the next thing you know, we started having sex and it was like every night. Do you want to calm down at least two, three days? Like rest for awhile.

The relationship lasted two months, and ended abruptly. Ethan described in detail why the relationship ended.

It ended when I introduced him to one of my friends. I introduced him to another hustler friend of mine named Jake. We had a three-way, Christopher paid Jake forty bucks, and Jake was going to leave. And Jake asks me, "Are you going to leave with me?" I said "No, I'm going to stay here with Christopher." Jake said, "Okay. Can I use your bathroom?" He asked Christopher, and Christopher said, "Yeah." Jake goes into the bathroom, and is in there for like an hour. I don't know what he was doing. We totally forgot that he was in there. We didn't hear Jake come out of the bathroom and leave. Jake took Christopher's wallet. Christopher got mad, and asked, "Why did your friend do that? Why did your friend rip me off?" I said I didn't know. He said, "For him to do that, that's going to put a really big dent in our friendship." Well, I said, "You know Christopher, I don't mean to sound like a bad guy. I don't want you to get the wrong idea, but I think our relationship has really gotten to a point where everything is just not on all four legs anymore. As far as what Jake did, when I run into him, I will speak to him." Christopher said, "When you run into Jake, ask him to bring my wallet back. He can keep the cash. All I want is my credit cards, my ID, my driver's license." I said "Okay." He was furious.

Ethan left, and he was again homeless and back on the street. He had been through similar situations, was resilient, and could quickly reconnect into sex-worker networks and life. He reestablished relationships with his friends, and stayed with former clients. He encountered Jake.

I asked him where Christopher's wallet was. He said "I don't know; I didn't take his wallet." I said, "Jake, why did you do that; I thought we were friends? You know Christopher asked me to ask one of my friends, to invite them to a small party. And right away I thought of you. I mean Christopher paid for the drugs. He paid for the cigarettes; he paid for the soda; he paid for the whole party. Why did you rip him off?" He says "blah, blah, blah." I said, "That's no excuse." The wallet was long gone. So I called Christopher and told him that Jake had kept the money and thrown his wallet away. I said, "Jake, apologize to Christopher." Jake says, "Okay." Jake says "Hi, how are you?" and Christopher starts yelling at him over the phone. Jake says (to Christopher), "You know what, you asshole, I'm fucking glad I ripped your fucking ass off. Fuck you," and hung up on him. I asked, "Why did you hang up on him?" "Because he called me a hustler; he called me a lowlife hustler. Forget that, I'm not going to take that. I'm glad that I ripped him off." I said "Well, Jake, do you know what you just did? You messed up something for me. I don't know if you realize this, but I was going out with this person, and I think you messed it up for us." He says, "I didn't mess it up for you; I just messed up for myself." He says, "I'll bet you anything that he is going to call you, or you're going to call him and he's going to say, 'yeah, come over.' He's going to like you more." Well, Jake was right; Christopher didn't really trip on me. It was Jake's fault. Jake did the crime.

Ethan continued to take money from Christopher, but did not live with him nor encourage reestablishing a relationship. In hindsight, he identified variations in relationships with johns and the psychological effects of these relationships on him over time.

In other words, you pay me to do something that you want me to do to you sexually, and I'll do it. But if I spend more than three days with you, I consider that something different. There's sex and then there's sex. There is sex for money, and there is sex because you like the person—that's the kind of sex that Christopher and I had. But after two or three years, four or five years of this, I became one big emotional wreck. I didn't know if this person loved me. I didn't know if this person liked me. I didn't know if this person wanted to have sex with me and just dump me–you know, give me money and not see me the next day. That was my little world, and I was real upset because I didn't like it. I didn't like the fact that I had to go to the streets to pull a trick and that I had to turn to this person for emotional help for anything.

Through 1989, Ethan continued to be a street regular, and spent most of his time with speed-addicted, sex-worker friends. He had enough of Northern California, and went back to Southern California to "cool out" for awhile. He saw an old friend.

I wasn't making any money on the street. I wasn't pulling any more tricks, because the tricks weren't interested in me, or I wasn't interested in them. Something didn't click, so I said "Well, okay, tonight I'll pull one trick and then I'm leaving. With that money, I'm taking the bus to go south." And that night I pulled that one trick; I went down to the bus station, I bought my ticket, and I left that night. I went south. That's when I saw Ray. I thought Ray had gone back east where his mother lived. He was driving down The Boulevard. He was driving a white Rolls Royce convertible, and he was looking real good. He had more cash on him this time then when he was in Northern California. He saw me and he said, "Hey, what are you doing down here?" He said, "Get in." "Ray, I'm trying to work." "Forget that, come on," he said. "Do you have a place to stay down here?" I said, "No, I'm trying to get some money so I can get a place." He said "Come on, you can stay at my place. . . . my hotel is paid up for two weeks." I said, "Okay, sure, I'll take it, why not?" So I went with him, and I stayed with him in his hotel. The day he drove me back to his hotel he gave me cash and some drugs, and he said, "If you want to go out you can go out. If you want to stay in you can stay in." He said he was going to sleep so he went to sleep. And I thought, "Well, now I have the cash so I don't have to go out now." So I stayed in and I watched TV and ate something, and nodded off. I went to sleep and I didn't realize that we slept all morning and all afternoon. . . . The next morning I woke up to pounding on the door. "This is the FBI." So Ray opened the door, and I got dressed. I came out of the bathroom. This one FBI person said to me, "I want you to get out." He pointed at Ray and said, "You are under arrest." And I said, "Why? This is my boyfriend. What are you doing?" He said, "Well, it seems your boyfriend has been stealing credit cards, and he's forging them. And you know that Rolls Royce you see out there? He stole that. That car has been reported stolen for two days." I'm thinking that everything that my friends were telling me back then was true. This guy is a fake, you know, and he gets me in trouble with the FBI. I said, "Ray, I don't know what to say other than I'm going back home. Thanks for the cash." The funny thing is that the FBI didn't know that Ray had cash. They didn't know that the cash was on me because they told me to leave, and I left. I had the cash. So I left with the hundred and fifty dollars. I took the next bus.

Ethan returned North, and "laid low." He stayed with his family for a week, but eventually returned to the streets he knew so well. He was aware of HIV and AIDS, and he would often take precautions to prevent infection. However, if the price was right, he would take the risk of infection. He recalled his price negotiations with one elderly customer.

Now him I did without a condom. But I told him "Don't come in my mouth." And he offered me fifty dollars to have oral sex. But I told him, "Look, I don't do it without condoms." He said, "Well, how about if I give you seventy-five dollars if we did it without a condom?" At that time I was desperate and I needed the money real bad. I said, "Well, okay. But don't come in my mouth. You come in my mouth, *that will be extra* money."

After four years of intermittent sex work including instances of unprotected receptive anal sex, and substance use including shared intravenous needle usage, Ethan tested HIV positive in 1989 at age 17. He was one of the first "chronically disenfranchised youths" known to service providers to test positive. He described how the notification was mishandled.

Well, at first I was a little scared because the nurse said that I was HIV positive. Then she said, "Oh, wrong tube." In other words, she had someone else's blood work. I said, "Well okay." So my blood work came in, and they said I'm negative. Then like a month later, positive. It hurt, like so I'm HIV positive. Everybody was really dramatic about it. "Oh, I'm HIV positive. Oh, I'm going to die two years from now." When I found out I thought, "Well, so, I'm HIV positive; what's next?" I mean what do you want me to do stand here and pout and cry over it? I'm HIV positive, and it has got its problems. Everybody is starting to worry about you because you don't look sick; you're not sick, but you are! It kind of complicates things with family, and friends, and work—whatever. It just separates you from life. But if you just look at it like, "Okay, I'm the same guy today." You take that and you go on with life. Don't worry about it. Don't even think about it. You know, if you feel like dying, then that's your choice. If you want to die, die. If you don't, go on with life!

His friend Jordan was the first person he told he had tested positive. Even though they had never been sexually intimate with each other, Jordan had many experiences in common with Ethan, and went to be tested soon thereafter. Ethan told his family about his infection, beginning with his mother.

She was scared. She said, "Well, my son can't be HIV positive. It's not like you see on television; it doesn't happen to my son." I told my mom being HIV positive can happen to anybody. "It's not your fault; it's not God's fault. It's nobody's fault. It's just a disease that we can't stop, but that we can prevent from happening to someone else." She looked at me and felt stupid. She said, "Like in the Bible, God says . . ." I said, "What does God have to do with this? God had nothing to do with this. God made the world—yes, I believe that. God made us—I do believe that too. But God didn't make this disease." . . . I told my sister about it. My sister, to this day, she still cries, "Oh God, you're HIV positive." She doesn't like it. She hates that I'm HIV positive.

His social worker arranged for a subsidized studio apartment for Ethan in 1993. The apartment was in a building in the downtown area and was occupied mostly by drug dealers, sex workers, and the elderly poor. The building had peeling yellow paint, dirty red carpets, and iron bars on the windows, and it was poorly lit. In Ethan's room, he had placed a mattress on the floor and had a portable radio near the window for entertainment. Clothes were scattered around the room, in places piled two feet high, like haystacks. These were used at times as chairs. There was no other furniture. Jordan lived across the hall, and Damian one flight up. Damian was a twenty-five-year-old "drag queen" who had been involved in the sex and drug scene since he was twelve. He was the parental figure of the group, the experienced elder and confidant of Ethan, Jordan, and Jared.

People were always coming and going, and Ethan sometimes allowed strangers without a place to stay to sleep at his place. He let twenty-three-year-old Sandy move in with him. She was an old friend, and like Ethan, a well-known speed dealer (middle person) in the area. She would at times trade sex for drugs, and she brought her sexual partners into Ethan's apartment. Other street friends would come over to use, buy, or sell drugs (or "product"). Sex-worker friends would bring clients and use Ethan's studio while they did their business. He had little privacy, and no room for introspection. Jared visited often, and would regularly stay overnight with Ethan or at Jordan's. There was a constant flow of people, or "drug traffic." Ethan had a telephone installed that everyone would use. The phone was employed to set up drug deals without having to leave the apartment. Eventually, Ethan could not pay the bill and the phone was disconnected.

Ethan spent Christmas Eve 1993 with Sandy, Jordan, Damian, and a couple of their friends. Together they ate, drank, and later danced all night in after-hours gay nightclubs.

> We were doing mushrooms and listening to the radio. There were about six or seven people in my house, two bottles of champagne, and two or three bags of mushrooms in a pot. Well, we just sat around and kind of spaced out off the Christmas tree. It wasn't standing in an erect position; it was leaning over. . . . It was actually the first time I spent Christmas with

friends. Like everybody came over and brought their own little thing. They brought their own food, a chocolate cherry cake; they brought like pies, and we just had a lot of food . . . . we were talking about five hundred ways how to kill a person, or ten men have a shoot out, or who's got the best dope.

To escape his apartment and friends, Ethan went to his mother's on Christmas Day, had dinner, and grudgingly answered all her questions about why he wasn't doing anything with his life. He returned to his apartment more depressed and began a speed run that would last until New Year's Eve. Other speed runs that followed for the next year usually extended up to six or seven days. During this time, Ethan rarely saw the morning, getting up around two in the afternoon. His daily routine was the same: he would rise, arrange drug deals, visit with friends, and go to The Program for free meals or to obtain medical or financial assistance. The late afternoon and evening were spent "tweaking" at home, at nightclubs dancing, or in sex work on the streets. If he was not on a speed run, he would go to sleep around 3:00 in the morning. The next day he would repeat the same activities, following approximately the same schedule. Along with Jordan, Damian, and Jared, Ethan was a regular and well known in the underground gay nightclub scene. Weekend participation in drug and nightclub activities were encouraged among the "crew."

> We go at 6:00 at night and hang out, get your hand stamped, and then go out and look for the people who are reported missing by other friends. We call it club sighting, get them altogether. You get them all drugged up, get them wasted, and take them to clubs.

Ethan's relationships facilitated good times, but were not particularly supportive or reliable. He had no lover or permanent sexual partner, even though he wanted one. He found it difficult discussing his specific homosexual activities with his male heterosexual social worker. Most of the people in his group of friends had tested HIV positive or were avoiding being tested. AIDS became a subject for humor in their conversations.

> When I'm at home, they're cracking jokes. They're saying I'm just going to die, die of AIDS and this and that. To me, when people say things like that, it's not funny. I don't find it funny. But somebody will say, "Oh, it is funny. You've got to live your life. Don't live your life so serious. You got to learn to take a joke every now and then." I've been taking jokes ever since I was a kid.

Clothing and other items routinely disappeared from Ethan's apartment only to "mysteriously" reappear later in Jordan's studio. Ethan claimed that Jordan and Sandy—or their friends—were stealing things from him and selling them or exchanging them for drugs. Verbal arguments and physical fights were frequent, but estrangements did not last long. The landlord of his building, even though profiting from the activities that occurred there, complained to Ethan's social worker about his sexual and drug-related activities. Sandy was forced out of the building, and eventually Ethan was evicted and moved into a hotel, an arrangement made by his social worker. The hotel was a good distance away from The Program office and from his friends. Ethan "hated" the hotel and didn't feel "safe." For the next few months, he lived in an even more "toxic environment."

> It was just the people I guess. There's all kinds of crack tools in the bathrooms when I went to shower. The shower was in the hallway, and when a person wanted to take a shower, they couldn't take a shower in a clean shower. It had burned matches and all kinds of stuff. At six o'clock in the morning, they would knock on my door—"Doesn't what's-his-name stay here?"—"No, he moved out." The prostitutes would bring in these guys off the streets, and pull dates. They did their job and then they would leave. Then they would come back with some other dude who you've seen in the alley like four million times, full of drugs. It just bothered me when they'd come knocking on my door looking for someone who didn't even live there, asking for all kinds of drugs.

With the help of his social worker, Ethan eventually found another apartment three blocks away from The Program. For a short period of time, he enjoyed the newfound privacy of having a room to himself. His previous illicit activities shifted to the new place, but in time became less frequent. The drug use and sex work continued, just at a slower, less frantic pace. Again, he let people who were "down and out" stay in his new apartment. These people served multiple purposes in his life. He described one as "like a boyfriend, a bed-buddy, and my dealer." He claimed it was "in his nature to take people in." He desired privacy, but the majority of the time he hated to be alone. For years, Ethan had lived for "pleasure." When on a speed run, he experienced a strong sexual drive, or "got the fevers."

> When I do a hit, it helps my sex drive, because as soon as you do it, a rush hits you, and your body starts tingling. It's a nice feeling, and it just hits you from the waist down. I get really horny, and I just have to go and take care of it. I go and take care of it. . . . In other words, it doesn't matter who, just so long as he's a man, or as long as he's a male.

Ethan went in the early hours of the morning to adult bookstores or traditional public male "cruising" sites.

> I haven't gone out much. I like to stay home. That's why I wish I had a boyfriend, or just had a relationship of some sort, where I can stay home. I think it's crazy having to go out sometimes and look for dick. After a while it gets boring. The only time I go to bookstores is when I've done too many hits, too many shots. I'm just up, mind out of control. That's the only place I can go and cum. It just hits you right there in your nuts. You get hot and bothered. You have to go there to be around something sexual; you have to be in a place where it's nothing but sex.

To quench his sexual desires and needs, he found additional ways to meet men.

> I used to go to this one office building and I'd get depressed. I would go there and I used to go in like their rest rooms. I would go there and I would have to go to the bathroom real

> bad. As I was walking around, it was driving me crazy. And I
> used to meet guys in the bathroom in these office buildings. It's
> like, "Hi, how are you? What's your name?". . . . There's a new
> person—I met him at the bank building.

When Ethan would meet a paying client, or a date from a club, the
topic of AIDS would sometimes enter into their presex discussions.
One representative example of a commercial sexual encounter is
given to illustrate how the topic of AIDS is both meaningful and
unimportant at the same time.

> That was the topic of the night. I told him that I was HIV
> positive. He said he was HIV negative. We listened to the radio
> and this girl came on and said she wanted to make a dedication
> to her boyfriend who had just died of AIDS. And I told him I
> did not want to hear that. And he said, "Why not?" And I said,
> "I just don't want to hear it. I hate people talking about people
> dying, people that they loved dying over the radio." He turned
> off the radio. That's when I told him that I was HIV positive.
> He didn't seem too excited. Well, he didn't seem like he really
> cared. I mean it's like he cared about the fact that I was HIV
> positive, but he didn't care about the fact that I was telling him
> this. . . . I was kissing him because I wanted him to know that
> that's how I am, and he doesn't have to take me back to his
> house. He can take me home if he wants. In other words, after
> I told him, I was leaving the decision up to him. If he wanted
> me to stay, that's fine; if he wanted me to go, that's fine too. He
> just looked at me and smiled and turned back on the radio. He
> said "Let's listen to some tunes." He put his arm around me,
> and he started talking, and then I kissed him. Kissing kind of
> expanded. We started kissing more and more and more, until
> we got to his house and then we started getting into it. . . . We
> did it on each other's chest, that was funny.

Through 1994, Ethan had many sexual encounters where he was
offered more money to have unsafe sex. If he refused, his fee was
sometimes involuntarily reduced. He continued to engage in all
varieties of homosexual activities with multiple partners and in public locations. He established short-term relationships with older

men, many in heterosexual marriages who for short periods of time would provide him with money or gifts. These customers would have the same unrealistic rescue fantasies of some service providers—that Ethan could quit sex work and drugs, and "go to college." Besides his sex work with older men, he would also have sexual liaisons or "tweak and freak" with men his own age, with "drag queens," with new youth in The Program, and with drug dealers in exchange for product, trading sex for drugs.

In late 1994, following a speed run, Damian, who had lived with HIV for years, committed suicide. Ethan had spoken with him the night before he died. Damian's death affected all of the members of his street-based family. The Program held a memorial service, which was well attended by staff and clients. Jordan went on a speed run and did not attend, instead "getting really wasted, just getting higher, and higher, and higher with no sleep." Ethan wanted to be sober for the memorial, and attended by himself. Damian's death moved him greatly. They had been close friends for over ten years.

> I think because Damian's death burned me. Ever since Damian's death, everything's changed. Me, my dopies, I mean my association with Jordan and Jared, I don't see them as often. . . . Damian and I had this agreement, if either one of us died, the one left would not carry on what the other person was doing, just the opposite. Damian's point was that he would do drugs and all the bad things, so I've got to do the opposite; I've got to stop doing drugs.

Ethan's resolve to quit drugs altogether did not last long, but he did curtail his use. He had more frequent contact with his mother and sister, visiting them on a more regular basis. Although he was twenty-three years old, and should have been transitioned to adult AIDS or social service programs, Ethan wanted to stay a Program client, and did not immediately transfer to adult AIDS or social service agencies.

> I just hate going through another organization, repeating what I've been doing here. I'd rather just stay here and have people take care of me.

In February 1995, his social worker tried to arrange an employment situation for Ethan in the Program's income-generating project. Ethan had never held a legitimate, regular job. As a teenager, he had worked at his mother's church bingo for a few months, and as a young adult, he had earned money as a middle man, and speed dealer. He continued in infrequent sex work, but had few if any other marketable skills. Generally healthy, with nonprogressive HIV, Ethan likely had many years ahead of him before the onset of AIDS or related disability. It was unclear whether he would ever voluntarily terminate the support of the social services system. His drug use and sex work decreased. He realized that his life was characterized by an undesirable routine. He wanted a change.

The same old thing every day. Wake up, shower and get dressed, get something to eat, come to The Program, get a food voucher and get something to eat, go back home and sleep, wake up at 5:30 in the evening, spend from 5:30 to 8:00 here at The Program, go back home, change clothes, go back out, find drugs, do drugs. It's like the same thing over and over and over. It's grueling. I just hope it ends.

Chapter 8

"Better and in a Different Way": Jared

*Thus in the intricate relations and graver circumstances of life,
there may often be found, associated with disappointment, a germ
of compensation.*

—Alexander Von Humboldt, *Aspects of Nature*, 1849

*The body, unclaimed after death, was turned over to a medical
college to be used in a classroom laboratory. The men who per-
formed the dissection were somewhat abashed by the body under
their knives. It seemed intended for some more August purpose, to
stand in a gallery of antique sculpture, touched only by light
through stillness and contemplation, for it had the nobility of some
broken Apollo that no one was likely to carve so purely again....But
death has never been much in the way of completion.*

Tennessee Williams, *One Hand*, 1948

Jared was twenty-three years old, white, bisexual, muscular, and
green-eyed, and had a warm, engaging personality. He was a friend
of Ethan's. He was extroverted and spontaneous in a carefree, fresh,
and youthful manner. His brown hair was straight, shoulder length,
and stylish, and he usually dressed in baggy, urban grunge wear. He
had been a model and a professional dancer, but remained shy and
somewhat unaffected by his physical attractiveness. While he was
streetwise and experienced, he still radiated an innocent, vulnerable
air. He claimed to be typical of Generation X.

Jared was born in the Eastern United States to parents of mixed
Italian/French and Portuguese/Puerto Rican backgrounds. His parents, both in their early twenties when he was born, had mainstream
jobs, but lived counter-cultural lives. He was allowed to do as he

pleased from an early age. He had two older brothers and an older sister, and one younger half-sister. His extended family included many "kinfolk" and aunts and uncles who played important but episodic roles in his life. He was a precocious child who never "did what everyone else did." He "wanted to do the opposite." He had his first sexual experience "under a bunk bed" at age nine with a thirteen-year-old female next-door neighbor; Jared remarked, "I've always been a little pervert, I guess." He tried marijuana for the first time at age ten. In his words, he grew up in "such a shady and creepy background," and he ran away from home at age eleven.

> I ran away. I got sick of the situations that were taking place and my parents were very, very heavy into cocaine, very heavy. They sold me out—that's all I have to say. Even at a young age, I knew. I've always been more, I don't want to say advanced, but more knowledgeable than people my age. Because knowledge is power, and I have one hell of a power trip. Them being how they were in their drug-induced psychosis—that's what I call it—and me being a smart aleck, I guess it just didn't work out. I was ready to go, and I just took off. . . . I was gone for a week just all over the city. I remembered where my friends lived and places that I'd visited because I had an excellent memory, so I could just get there. And then all these things just happened; I don't know how they happened, or why they happened, why I took off. I understand my reasoning behind it, but how I did it at such a young age. . . . The reason that I left home, the reason that I did all these things and stayed away from home is because of who they were, and not because I didn't want to have a home. See, I don't know how to explain it without—Jesus, I must sound like a nut.

According to Jared, he always looked older than his age and did things that youths his age did not know how to do. His recollections at times seemed fantastic, but the experiences he claimed to have had in early adolescence were recalled in detail and repeatedly over time. At age twelve he went with a friend and her family to Europe, ran away from this family, and eventually lived with squatters for a year and a half. "It was easy because people live on the streets there, like I grew up in this. I was a punk rocker, and I grew up." He lied about his age and got a job in a stockroom in a large department store. His parents discovered that he ran away after arriving in Europe because he did not want to return to them. According to Jared, they gave up on him and made no attempts to locate him.

At age twelve, Jared had his next sexual experience, which included active and receptive oral sexual activity with his male supervisor at work.

> That was my introduction into bisexuality. It was fun, but the encounters I had over there were far and few between. Because, especially the punk rock crowd, they shun sex. They think it's a gross American thing. It's very mental, and music, and your relationship–it's not physical. . . . The first time I ever had sex was at the department store, as a matter of fact with my boss. He was nineteen. He was a punk rocker. I'd always had an interest in it. See, I guess I find everything that's like wrong, fascinating. I want to know why, why is it wrong? And then if I do it, can I make a right way to do it? So I thought, "I'll try anything once," and so I did. It was fun because it was so wrong. It wasn't the actual doing it, it was the rush from it, I guess the taboo. . . . I've always known things I guess. I mean nobody has ever really taught me, this is how you give a blow job, or this is how you do this, or this is how you do that. I don't know why, but I've just always known things. Of course I've heard people talk about things, I'm sure, and picked up things, but I really can't explain how I knew what to do. It just came natural. I've always been a fag [laughs]. I just like to sleep with beautiful people. I have no color, sex, or sexuality preference. I had sex with a black guy for the first time on my birthday. I was at a gay bar, but at that time it was unisex; you know, anybody could go. Homosexual or heterosexual, nobody cared. How you dressed, nobody cared, because they were there for one thing, for the music, to dance, period.

Dancing was a major way Jared expressed himself. Regulars in the club scene accepted all forms of sexual activity, homosexual or heterosexual. He tried ecstasy and smoked heroin for the first time. After a year and a half of living in squats and on the streets in Europe and without money from age fourteen, Jared contacted his parents and with their help, returned to the United States. Because of past difficulties, instead of returning to live with his parents, Jared went to live with an uncle and aunt in the South. Both were in their early forties. Jared had lived a fast life for two years in Europe, and returned to live in the slower paced, conservative, rural South. His uncle and aunt were more like friends to Jared, rather than limit-setting adults or parental substitutes. They treated him fairly, respected his privacy, and gave him a job on the dude ranch they managed. He was able to earn and save money working at the ranch, and he made "extra money" helping his uncle and aunt in their side business, growing marijuana. Even though he had no formal schooling while in Europe, he had spent a lot of his free time in libraries and reading. Self-taught, and surprisingly well-read, Jared was able to attend high school in the South. He stood out from other students, and his good looks, charm, and social skills served him well.

> I was popular with all different types of groups, the nerds, preps, the jocks, everyone. I never had one specific group of friends. I was always the weirdo, though, because I was a punk rocker. When I first arrived I had a purple Mohawk, dressed in army fatigues, and my nose was pierced. . . . Those hillbillies flipped out. I gave those children hell. . . . I played football; I was on the dive team; I played basketball. I did everything that a regular kid would do, but *better and in a different way.*

Jared recalled that people were intrigued by his punk rocker appearance—"guys hit on that a lot." He was openly bisexual in high school and was "hit on" by "straight guys, guys with wives, my friends' parents—like fathers." He remembered having separate sexual liaisons with his best friend's thirty-eight-year-old father and mother.

> One day we were bailing hay. My friend was sick and so I was helping his father. We were bailing hay, and I went to take a piss, and he was like pissing down from me; I was looking over and talking to him. I said something, and he said something else. He said, "Do you want to do something." I said, "Yes," and I did it [oral sex]. I mean it wasn't like I had ever really dreamed about it. Because he asked me, I did. Because it was spontaneous I guess. . . . His (Jared's friend's) mother, she

was always flirting with everybody. She was a Southern belle. She was a wild woman in town. Flirty. . . she would always hit on me, joking around. That was just her personality. I was tired of her talking about it, so I made her do it one day. That was it. I told her to shut up and do it. "I'm sick of hearing you say it–do it." We had oral sex and intercourse.

Even though sexual activities occurred only once with his friend's parents, all three remained silent about the incidents. Jared, however, retained respect for his friend's father.

> I respected him a lot, because he was quite the man, very much the stud, a good-old boy. But we never discussed it. It was like, "Okay, we did it, it was hot" and that was it. It was like it never happened, that kind of thing. . . . She made an issue of it, without saying a word. She felt very guilty I think. She was very withdrawn toward me, and I didn't understand it. I had a hard time with that.

His friend's father was the last man Jared had sexual contact with until he was eighteen. The third summer he lived in the South, Jared went on vacation and met and had a sexual affair with Jenny. They became very close, and were "soul mates" in Jared's words. Eventually, Jenny became pregnant. She initially told Jared she would have an abortion. She soon changed her mind, decided to go through with the pregnancy, and gave birth to a son. Shortly after she found out she was pregnant, she invited another boyfriend to live with her. He raised the boy as if it were his own child. This boyfriend knew the baby was not his, but Jared's.

Following high school graduation and soon after he returned from vacation, Jared left the South and came to California to stay with another aunt, who he discovered was bisexual. His sexual activity was never a topic of conversation with his aunt, since "she never paid that much attention" to him anyway. In California, he was introduced to Brad, his aunt's middle-aged, gay, male friend who educated him on gay life and community. Brad was Jared's first contact with the gay world, and eventually proved his first direct experience with AIDS.

He showed me around, showed me where the clubs were if I wanted to go, or when I'd come down to visit, I'd stay at his house. When I did start getting into the club scene and things, he gave me insights. . . . He died of AIDS; my aunt and I took care of him. As a matter of fact, he died smoking a joint with me.

Shortly after coming to California, Jared went to live with a third aunt in a rural suburb. At age eighteen, he found a job in a retail store and established his own apartment in a nearby community. He often came into the city and danced in trendy nightclubs. Initially, Jared did not limit his sexual activities to either women or men. He "kept his options open."

My sexuality's always been open, always. If somebody said, "Look at that girl," and there was a guy with that girl, I'd say, "Both of them are hot; I'd do them both." . . . If a guy hit on me, a guy or a girl, I'm the same way. It's like it would be if you were straight and a girl hit on you, and you wanted to have sex with her; it was just like that. Except for me it was a guy or a girl; it didn't matter to me.

Jared went through periods during which he had more sex with women than men. Eventually, he had sex predominantly with men. His rationale for this change reflected more on his character than on his sexuality.

Well, I prefer men more now. I don't know why. I guess it turns me on more. It's more intense. I love the battle of ego. That turns me on so much. You use your head more in the gay life than you do in the straight life. As far as men, men are always trying to be one step ahead of each other, to be the more macho, the testosterone thing.

At age eighteen, working and living in a rural suburb, Jared met his first lover at the mall where he worked.

He was going up the escalator, and I was on a break. I went up the escalator, and God, this is so embarrassing. He went into

the bathroom. I went to the bathroom, and we met there. Then
it progressed [laughs].

Jared gave the twenty-three-year-old stranger "head" (oral sex) in a
bathroom stall. Later he spent nine months living with him, and
engaged in receptive anal intercourse for the first time. He wavered
on whether he believed the relationship involved love or not.

> I've never really experienced love before, I'd never loved
> anybody. Because I never let myself get close to anybody
> before. He was really the first that I did. I've always been a
> none-of-your-business kind of person; I'll do what I want, but
> you'll know nothing about me. He was my first; yeah, he was
> my first–I thought I was in love, but I wasn't. . . . I was doing
> everything for the wrong reasons, because that's what people
> do when they think they love each other, trying to live up to the
> stereotype of what love is. I would have all the want and
> desires of the other, but I pretended that was what I wanted. It
> was awful. It was my place; he moved in. He still had his own
> place where he could go, but he was always with me. He had
> another place; he just never used it. . . . When I met him, I
> freaked out, cause I thought I was in love with a guy; I was
> tripping out. I came home, I was sitting on the bed, and I
> flipped out for some reason. "My God, I'm gay!" I tripped
> out. I never thought about it before. I'd always done things; I'd
> just never really thought about them because they were no big
> deal to me. And then I thought about it and I was, "Oh wow! I
> think I love him; Jesus, what's happening to me?" I'd never
> thought about things the way that others do. I fucked with my
> friend's mom and dad and didn't care less. It was like picking
> my teeth with a toothpick and throwing it out. I didn't care
> [laughs]; it wasn't any big deal to me, and I never thought
> about it.

Jared, with his closest friends Jordan, Ethan, and Damian, spent
most of his free time either using speed or dancing at gay and
lesbian nightclubs. Even though Jared lived in a rural area, he frequently came into the city to "party." Jordan and Ethan had been

either homeless or in unstable housing situations for years, and were known in the gay, adolescent, sex and drug street worlds.

> We are the only family that each other has, and no matter how many times we've messed each other over, there's a love established that can't be killed.

Jordan had a crush on Jared since they first met, but their relationship never involved sexual activity. Jared had oral sex with Ethan on one occasion, the only time Jared claimed to have sex with someone from the "crew."

> We all play around, you know. You know how guys are, girls are too, when they're all together in their room they sort of like, "Oh baby," da-da-da-da-da. He started rubbing my thigh, and things went from there. It didn't change things in a negative way. If anything, we had another experience under our belt that's close and intimate.

Jared and his friends routinely went to the nightclubs early to avoid paying the entrance cover charge. On weekends, he went out at 9:00 p.m. on Saturday evenings and danced from after-hours club to after-hours club into Sunday afternoon. He danced for hours nonstop, "I don't even stop to use the restroom." He described his typical behavior in clubs.

> I dance by myself. I meet people, but it's "Oh, hi, how you doing? I'm going to dance." I'd take off and start dancing again. Usually when I go to a club, I don't really go in there to scope on anybody. I usually don't talk to anybody unless they come up to me when I am on the dance floor. I mean that's where I am the whole time, from the minute I walk in to the minute I leave.

Jordan introduced Jared to his housemate, Asher, and they started a relationship that lasted for two years. Jared had seen Asher in clubs and in gay neighborhoods before. Asher was six years older than Jared and worked in a mansion as a live-in caretaker. He was also a high-level drug dealer. Jared eventually realized that Asher was also "a hard-core speed freak." Asher had been a sex worker in his adolescence and early twenties and was a regular on the streets. Jared described Asher as intelligent, and a "hard-core case of addictive-compulsive personality." He explained his attraction to Asher.

> He was real mysterious. He was a bad boy, you know. I mean he was a really bad, bad boy, troublemaker. He's tough. He's all the things that people shouldn't be. I'm attracted to the darker side I guess. He's the sexiest man I've ever met in my life.

Jared moved into the mansion and paid Asher $350 for a month's rent. Asher was not allowed to have others living in the mansion with him, but frequently let "street regulars" crash there when they needed a place to stay. Jordan, for example, had been living there for a month in between times he spent with lovers or friends. The first night in the mansion, Jared snorted speed. By the second night, Jared and Asher were no longer just roommates but became intimate sexual partners. After the first month, Jared started living in the mansion rent-free.

> Two days later, we were all really messed up. Asher was there, and I was in my room. He came in, and was talking to me, and one thing led to another. We had sex. . . . It was many, many things. It was very hot, very passionate. It's the kind of thing that when you cum, you cry. There was something there; we could feel it. We fell asleep.

When Jared and Asher had anal sex that night, Jared was the insertive partner. They slept with each other from that night on. After three months, they tried reversing anal sexual roles. In their subsequent sexual activities, both took oral receptive and insertive roles. Asher frequently ejaculated in Jared's mouth, and Jared swallowed the ejaculate.

During the initial months he lived in the mansion, Jared did part-time modeling for department stores, and he earned substantial money for print advertisements that ran in local papers. However, the modeling work was not consistent, and the money was quickly spent. Asher received a small salary for his caretaker duties and would also earn money through his drug dealing, or unknown to Jared at the time, for sexual services with clients from his "younger days." Most of his friends, including Jordan and Ethan, used speed intravenously, or "slammed." Jared, who had previously only snorted speed, shot up with Asher using separate needles. He suspected Asher was HIV infected. When Jordan moved out, Jared and Asher's sexual relationship intensified. In time, they stopped using condoms altogether.

> We used condoms up until, like a month after we started sleeping together. Then it was like, you know, well. Until the AIDS test and we went and had an AIDS test together. We both came out negative.

They tested for HIV together because Jared knew Asher's past drug and sexual history. He was concerned that Asher was infected, and wanted to "start fresh," and live as a monogamous couple. Jared, wanting to please Asher, suggested that they reverse their anal sex roles.

> I said, "I don't think it's fair that I get to do it to you all the time, and knowing how much you like to do it–do you want to try?" But there was no way. I can't relax enough to have it done. . . . We tried it and it didn't work. It hurt too much. I couldn't do it. He didn't want to do it because it hurt me. I always heard that it hurt at first and then you get used to it, so I was taking pain. But like the second time after we did it, I started bleeding when I had a bowel movement, really bad, like for two days. I had to go to the doctor. I never tried it again after that.

In time, Jared discovered that Asher was having sexual relations with other men. Although the trust between them ended, they remained together because Jared thought, "You were supposed to put up with a lot, that was what you were supposed to do when you were in love." Jared eventually got on the mansion payroll by doing gardening and maintenance work. Asher was arrested for drug dealing and was sent to jail. Jared took care of the mansion by himself until Asher's return. The mansion was eventually sold, and they moved together to a "gay" area in Southern California. The relationship ended there, and Jared found his own apartment. They continued to see each other daily. A few months later Asher was arrested for grand theft auto and went to prison.

Jared returned to Northern California and immediately located his old street friends, including Ethan and Jordan, through The Program. Ethan was slamming more speed than before and was involved in more sex work in order to maintain his drug habit. Jared engaged in sexual activity for money only on a few occasions.

> I only did it three times. I can't take it. I can't take it. I feel so guilty doing it. I feel guilty. I feel it degrades me to do it. Sex for money, that kind of thing. It's me and that weird sex thing again.

One of his former "tricks" was a forty-seven-year-old former minister from whom he sought advice whenever he had problems. The man was living with HIV, and had lost his lover to AIDS. Most of Jared's casual or street friends, including Ethan, were active sex workers. He described the effects that sex work had on people in negative and strongly judgmental terms.

> I don't like what it represents. I think it is disgusting. Look what it does to people. You have to see it firsthand. It brings them down. I mean they turn into IV-shooting, disrespectful, dishonest sluts. That's all they are. I had a choice whether I wanted to do it or not, and I chose not to. There are some of us who are just too stupid, others who don't have enough self-respect, those who don't have any other choice, and then there are those who just don't give a damn.

Even though he was forced to live with friends in sex-worker and drug-saturated environments, Jared tried to spend time with friends who were not actively involved in sex-work or street-drug worlds. For the past four years, he had a close relationship with a lesbian couple, Amanda and Bev. Originally, Jared had a sexual relationship with Amanda, a striking, blond college student. In time, he had sexual relations with both Amanda and Bev.

> I have a lot of friends who are lesbians. At the Cheese Pot, Club Snatch, I go hang out with them. I don't go to clubs to

pick up people, so it's mainly for the dancing, and they have good music. It's pretty much established I'm not there to scam. I'm a fag, and I'm just there to dance.

When Jared slept with both Amanda and Bev, they had oral and insertive vaginal sex with condoms. Amanda and Bev decided they wanted a child. They discussed the possibility of Jared impregnating Amanda and marrying her, and the couple living with Bev as an extended family with an eventual male partner to be found for Jared. Worried that he might be HIV infected and not wanting to infect Amanda, Jared scheduled an HIV test at The Program where Jordan and Ethan were already clients. Jared had accompanied them to The Program on a number of occasions for food and financial assistance. He was already well-known by the staff as one of the long-term "chronic kids" and "crew members" who had lived a "marginal, unconnected life" for years.

In May 1993, Jared was tested for HIV a second time at a community-based STD clinic. He tested negative. The week after he tested and before he obtained the results, he went with his friend Matt to a sex club/bathhouse. There he met his next lover, twenty-two-year-old Aaron. His recollections are quoted in detail.

I'd never been there before, and my friend took me, and left me there. I was stuck there for sixteen hours. We went early Sunday morning, or Sunday going into Monday. . . . I had met Matt; he'd just gotten back from a party, and I was on my way back home. He was at a drugstore, so I followed him in there. I was talking to him, and he asked if I wanted to go with him? "Oh, sure." I thought I was going to help him move some stuff out of a storage locker, even though it was late. I mean he's a tweaker, so he does that kind of stuff, and he said, "No we're going to the bathhouse." "What's that?" And he told me. I said, "Oh, cool." I thought it was going to be really gross; it was really clean. . . . I walked in, got my room, and I fell asleep for like the first four hours—went into my room and locked the door and I was sleeping. I woke up and this guy was going into the room next door. He said "Hey, how you doing?" and I said, "Okay, how you doing?" This boy was too much. He was really, really hot. He's Mediterranean. I went there at 4:30, so this was about 8:30 Monday morning. I said I was going to work out, we talked for a minute, and I went into the gym. I walked around with a baseball cap, my combat boots, and nothing else but a towel. He said, "God, you snore loud." He could hear me snoring because the rooms have no ceiling on them. I thought to myself, "God, idiot, snatch him now." I was working out and he came in. He said, "Do you mind if I work out with you?" I said, "No." One thing led to another, and I was laying on the bench doing curls, inverts. There were mirrors, the whole place was mirrored, and I was lying on the bench with only a towel doing inverts. I looked and I could see that he was staring at me in the mirror. And I was so horny, I started to get an erection. Well, he reached down and grabbed it, and I looked at him, and I just continued to work out. . . . We went and took a shower, went to the steam room went into the jacuzzi, went back into the steam room, and then I asked him if he wanted to come back to my room.

It was Aaron's twenty-second birthday. Jared bought three hits of ecstasy as a "sort of birthday gift" from a dealer he recognized in the bathhouse, and they both got "wired." Through conversation, Jared learned that Aaron lived with his parents, was a student, worked in a restaurant, sold marijuana for extra income, and had a girlfriend he "loved." Aaron had served in the military, during the Gulf War. Jared was impressed. Jared described how the drugs took effect.

> We were talking, listening to music. It took about a half an hour or forty-five minutes to kick in. But it was really hot in the building, so your blood's really speeding up. I said to him, "I want to go take a shower real quick, because I'm really hot." I went into the sauna room and all of a sudden, I just started going, oh-oh-oh. I started laughing, because it started kicking in. It tickled all over, and our rooms were really close to the showers and sauna. He could hear me laughing, and he came in and he was laughing too. I said, "I have to get out of here; I'm really full, really, really, high."

Involuntary muscle contractions followed, and both Jared and Aaron began to have body spasms. Jared had never done a hit and a half of ecstasy before, and he felt like a "mess." Shortly thereafter, the oral and anal sex began and continued for eight hours.

> I'd never, ever, ever, ever, and Asher is the only person who ever entered me ever. I liked this guy. It wasn't just that I was high; I felt really comfortable with him and I liked his energy and he was like intelligent, for someone my age. He drives a nice car, he goes to school, he's just right on. I had a really good feeling about him. The whole time I was talking to him I just wanted to like reach over and kiss him, and I'm not an affectionate person at all. This was even before I got high. He liked it very much because he kissed me back. I hadn't had sex with a guy in a long time. It was so hot. We were laying down, and the sheets, there was actually a puddle on the mattress, it was so hot. We were rolling. Have you ever met somebody and you're so into them, and they're so into you, that you roll around and it's like playing football in bed. . . . I went inside him. . . . We had oral sex, got up, and took showers. I mean I came nine times. Every time we'd cum, we'd get up and take a shower and then run back to the room. It was the most incredible sex I've ever had in my life, ever.

They ran out of money, and left the bathhouse late in the afternoon. Matt had already left, and Aaron drove Jared back home. Aaron stayed with Jared that night. Aaron called in sick at work the next day, and they spent the entire day together dining in an elegant restaurant and exploring the coast. That night, Jared had to prepare for a job the next day choreographing and cage-dancing at the opening of a large gay nightclub. Aaron accompanied him to rehearsal, and they had oral sex in the club office during breaks. For the next five months Jared and Aaron had a torrid relationship. However, the same week, after he had sex with Aaron, Jared also had sex with Amanda and Bev. He described how he experienced "the difference."

> It's different. I mean, how it is to have sex with a woman and how it is to have sex with a guy. One is like religion, the other is like being a blasphemer. It's like the difference between heaven and hell. One is really nurturing and compas-

sionate and tender; that hyper is still there, but it's controlled with a woman. With a guy, it's like, pow, pow, pow! It's thunder!

Jared retrospectively explained how his sexual preference and self-identity were not identical, and how his relationship with Aaron and Aaron's parents developed.

> We went back to his house. Aaron said, "You opened my eyes to a whole new world. I don't see gay as dirty and nasty and a bunch of queens and everything." He's said, "You're the coolest gay guy I've ever met in my entire life." I said, "I'm not gay; I'm just myself. I do whatever I want to do, and I don't make anybody pay the price for it. Just because you do something behind a closed door with somebody sexually does not mean that you are a stereotypical gay person—homosexual. If you live that lifestyle, then you are gay. You are a fag. If you act like a fag, then that's what you are. I don't choose to live like a fag, and I don't choose to live my life in the gay lifestyle per se. I have gay friends and I partake in activities, my life isn't all gay." He said, "Oh, I think that is so cool, and that's so hot." We both went and got our noses pierced as a symbol of being together. We went to his house, and he told his mom about me, and I met his mom and dad. They're hard-core about religion like my family, and they were kind of weird at first. But, I have a way of breaking the ice with people like that. His mom loves me, and his dad is really cool with me. I mean, I helped his dad rebuild a carburetor and a bunch of different things. I spent some time with them.

During the next few months Jared and Aaron house-sat or lived with friends, most of whom were drug dealers, substance users, or sex workers. Jared learned that Aaron had received a dishonorable discharge for smoking crack while in the armed services. As a couple, on a "honeymoon," they traveled north to visit Jared's aunts, and continued on a two-week camping trip, selling and dropping acid as they went along.

> We had a stash. We bought one hundred hits of acid, a sheet for forty dollars. Vampire Trance is what it's called. It was the

most killer experience I have had in my entire life. When I was tripping, we were out in the middle of the woods. We were eight miles into the middle of the wilderness. Nowhere, there was no one around. Running water, four or five different wading pools, and stuff like that, waterfalls, animals all around. It was great. We tripped our asses off. I climbed trees. I love to be in the woods and nature more than I do in the city. That's where I'm at peace. For the first four days I was totally sober. He was wigging out on acid and stuff like that; it was fun and everything. I wanted to try it. Sometimes when Aaron and I would be laying together, and he would reach over and put his arm around me, I would trip out on the inside. I would think [whispers], "This is a guy; what is God thinking!" I tripped off on it. I didn't care. God has seen me do some weird shit.

Jared, who had experimented with most street drugs, and was expert on street pharmacopoeia, described the effects that speed and acid had on him.

Speed, crystal's an evil drug because I always had a sex drive from hell, you know what I mean—sober or not. I don't have a sex drive like I used to before, maybe because I'm getting older. I don't have that grrrrrr that I used to, sober. As soon as I do speed, I could bust out of prison, it gets that intense. Acid, I trip off it like nobody else. I'm a lightweight in the first place. I can do less than everyone else, be messed up for longer and be higher, and have more fun for some reason. I use my imagination. With acid, I could be in the middle of having sex and everything could be great. Then one thing distracts me, and it's all blown until the next wave of the peak comes. Then it's sexual again, and then something else will distract me. Like to the point of a bird singing. Like these crows when we were camping were going caw, caw, caw, and I was tripping so hard they were distracting me. And we were in the middle of having sex, and making out in the middle of the woods. I didn't wear clothes for two weeks. I loved it. I climbed trees naked. It was great. I'm like a total nudist at heart anyway.

A few months later, they went on another trip together attending a rock concert. On the second trip, hallucinogenic mushrooms and marijuana were their drugs of choice. Jared differentiated between the effects that chemically produced versus more natural substances had upon him.

> I'm a nature freak, herbs and stuff like that. . . . Acid, crystal, ecstasy, all are chemical highs. That messes with me really bad. I can't be totally comfortable with it. If I'm tripping on mushrooms or on pot, I'm myself completely, one hundred percent. I've been smoking pot since I was ten years old. . . . I forget what my point was.

Aaron's drug use and resulting paranoia and jealousy limited their activities as a couple. Jared stopped seeing his friends and dancing at clubs. When Aaron wanted to try injecting or slamming speed, Jared felt that the end of the relationship was near.

> He said, "I want to try it sometime. I want to know how it feels. I just want to try it once." I said, "Aaron, you're an addictive, compulsive personality just like I am. There's no sense in trying it. Please, I love you too much. If you do we can't be together, because I know where it will lead and I can't have that in my life. I just got over that and if you can't understand that maybe we should just walk away now, or lessen the load and be friends and not lovers." He said, "I love you baby, and I won't do it duh, duh, duh." Well he pissed me off. It was just too much, we spent twenty four/seven every single day together. . . . I was never proud of slamming, and if people would ask me, I would always deny it.

In September of 1993, Jared packed up a pair of shorts, four T-shirts, a jacket, and a bottle of cologne in his backpack and left. The previous month he had gone to the Metaphysical Center where he was training to be a medium. He had his past lives charted, and bought thirteen decks of Tarot cards. When he left Aaron, he left a number of things behind, including the Tarot cards, which were "very, very important" to him.

> I left him. It's really hard because I've been running speed all my life, and he at times is a drug dealer on the side, and a

drug dealer that can't handle his product. When he does it, he gets in psychosis beyond belief. Paranoid, he accused me of setting him up, of cheating on him, cutting the wires on his car. . . . He turned out to be everything I was avoiding. The reason I liked him was because all of the people I met were tweakers and nasty. They had no couth about themselves; drugs were like their whole life. He seemed like just a part-time partier, and like he had his stuff together. He had a really nice car. He took care of himself–clean nails are really important. If I meet somebody with clean nails, it's really unusual.

Jared wrote a poem in his daily planner after leaving Aaron to express how the love they shared had changed:

> Where's the object that I gave the name love
> How is it something so powerful
> Strong enough to be called emotion
> Could lessen those emerging from intuition
> Could quickly fade from the eye
> Blink by Blink.

Just before his relationship with Aaron ended, a family crisis forced Jared to deal with issues in his life he had been avoiding. His younger half-sister, whom he barely knew, had to have a kidney transplant. According to Jared, "She and I are the only ones who have the same type of blood, and I guess it's a big factor." His family, who had "abandoned him," wanted him to donate a kidney. He told his mother he would have to consider it, and get back to her. Until the time when this request came, Jared had not spoken with his family for over a year. One week later he called his mother back. He made sure not to use very many mind-altering substances before he made the phone call. He described the rationale for this decision.

I haven't used any since Friday. I was trying not to use as much so I could get my shit together, so I'm not like high and coming down and lazy and saying, "Oh, no, I'll take care of that tomorrow." I wanted to be able to deal with things with a clear head. I figured with something this serious, and the things I had to deal with in my life right now, the best thing to do is to

be clean and sober when I deal with them. Because I've dealt
with so many things that were important like this, messed up,
and look at the outcome. I'm still in a weird predicament,
without a living space and a job and everything like that. If I
deal with things as they come along, clean and sober, they
seem to work out better in the end. And, I can remember what
people say.

Given his past sexual and drug use activities, he was hesitant to
make any commitments to his family. In the past year, he had
learned that Asher had seroconverted HIV positive. Jared re-created
his last phone conversation with his mother and how he shared his
concerns.

I haven't had an AIDS test in a while and the last one I had
was negative. I told you about my ex-lover saying that he was
positive, and it's possible that I am, too. I have to find out all
that first. I've shot speed; I've partied a lot; my blood isn't
going to be healthy for her. . . . I let them have it with the truth,
that I'd shot drugs, that I was gay, and I'd had unsafe sex with
somebody who was HIV positive, and that the conditions that I
live my life under weren't healthy enough to give the kidney. I
didn't appreciate their putting me in that position, by asking.
They hung up on me.

He did not hear from them again.

In the Spring of 1994, Jared tested again for HIV at The Program,
where Ethan and Jordan were already receiving HIV-related services. In hindsight and reflecting on the possibility he was positive,
Jared related his feelings toward Asher.

I don't have any anger toward him. I knew my risks, and I
did it anyway. The heat of the moment, I guess, or being high,
and still having love for him. If it were going to come up in the
test that I am positive, It's not going be like, "Oh my God,"
and that kind of thing. I've had friends all around me–Ethan,
Jordan, all my closest friends have it. It wouldn't be a big deal
to me. My social worker asked me, "Do you want to be positive?" "No! Why would I want to be positive?" That's like

saying, "Yes, I want to die." I don't want to die; I like my life. I mean as tough as it is, and as shitty as it is sometimes, as much as I've learned, I like it. Just because I'm positive it's not going to stop. As a matter of fact, it would give me the drive to go even further. There's no three-letter word, or four-letter word, disease or cold or whatever it is, I can't even see, bring me down. I've been through too much. The only three letter word that's going to get me is G-O-D, you know. I'm not going to trip off on it. I'm not afraid of it.

He tested HIV positive.

The only thing I wanted to know was "Is it AIDS or is it HIV?" It's HIV. And actually, it doesn't trip me out that much. I think because I was prepared by watching my friends and taking care of people. I know for sure now.

Jared's biggest concern became how and when he would tell Aaron. They had engaged in unprotected oral and anal sex, and Aaron had been at different times both the insertive and receptive partner.

My biggest thing with it is not myself, it's telling him about it. He's going to flip out. My social worker told me the possibilities of him being positive from just . . . coming in his mouth are a lot slimmer. What's really weird, he used to ask me all the time to cum in him. I wouldn't do it, and I don't know why. Maybe like somewhere subconsciously I was trying to protect him, could that be?. . . . I have to tell him, I owe him that. I can't live with myself if I don't. I would expect or would hope that someone would do that for me. I mean that's the responsible thing to do.

By the summer of 1994, Jared had enough of the drug and sex scene and left to be with less "toxic" friends. Jared's T cells were in the 1,100 range, and an AIDS diagnosis was probably years away. According to his case manager, by early 1995, he was active in an alternative religious cult and had moved into their rural commune. Jared evolved from child runaway in the Eastern United States, to adolescent squatter in Europe, to dancer and drug user in California, to young-adult truth seeker in a religious commune in the Southwest. The pattern and direction of his life was unclear to him. He had traveled far in search of internal peace, love, happiness, and stability. At the end of one interview, Jared revealed his desire to develop a self-empowering consciousness and confidence while he recognized his avoidance of retrospection and introspection.

See, I don't know how to explain a lot of the things I did, like the experiences and stuff. Because I don't think about them. I did them, and then moved on. I really don't think about why; I really don't think about it. Is that bizarre to not think about things? I just do them; it comes naturally. I do it and I go on. I don't dwell on it. I'm recalling all these things–I sometimes feel crazy because of that, because I really don't even think of them as memories. They just happened. That's it and move on. Is that strange? When I talk to people sometimes, they say "You mean you don't think about your parents? You don't think about this?" "No. Why?" All I'd do is sit around and be bummed out the whole time about it. I mean, I realize it's in existence and all, but I don't think about things, I put them on the back burner. . . . I'm tripping out about a lot of things in myself, and that's one of them. I almost can't remember my past. I've just pushed it all out of my head. I mean I did it, that's it, bye. My mind won't let me recall the memory. I get a block there because I don't think about it. I don't tell anybody my life. I don't tell anybody my business, period. You'll hear only up to a certain point, and you'll be satisfied, and when the door closes, you will know too [laughs]. I leave it that way because I don't want to talk about it. I don't want to think about it. I just don't think about it. For me to be sitting here discussing it, verbalizing it, is very hard for me, very awkward. It's very strange for me to be doing this because it meant a lot to me. I was affected more deeply by the things that happened to me when I was growing up, that we've talked about, that we got into. They hurt me a lot–a lot–and made me that very untouchy, unemotional person, kind of cold. I'm starting to get emotional about it; I don't want to feel the pain by even thinking about it, so I don't. You'll know more about me by the time that this is over than anybody I've come in contact with, probably since I was fourteen. Nobody, I mean, it's really weird. It's been kind of lonely too, to tell you the truth.

Before leaving California, Jared had a long talk with Jordan. Their friendship had been strained for some time.

I've told Jordan, "I said, I'm trying to go up and if you're going to stay stuck and stagnant, I'll drop you out of my life because it doesn't work having you as a friend. I care about you too much, and I have too much fun with you, getting high and fucking up and doing whatever we do. The only way I'm going to go up–is to be away.

In January 1995, Jordan took a bus to see Jared. Jared was supposed to meet Jordan at the bus station. Jared never came, and Jordan returned to California dejected. Jared changed his mind and didn't want to see his old "speed-running partner." He wanted to leave Jordan and other parts of his past behind.

Chapter 9

"Use the System to my Advantage": Lisa

Thou shalt go down to him to console the shades,
Thy youth shall be a light to their distress,
Thy spring shall charm away their everlasting winter,
Come, Thou shalt be queen of the shades.

          –Andre Gide, *Persephone*, 1949

For me neither the honey nor the bees.

          –Sappho of Lesbos (In Weigall, 1937)

Lisa was a twenty-four-year-old, street- and agency-smart lesbian from the Pacific Northwest. She was petite, but athletic, with long, dark brown hair, and large, expressive, brown eyes. She wore tight-fitting clothing, accentuating her figure. She was especially bright, confident, outspoken, and opinionated. Her mother abandoned her and her older brother and sister, leaving them with their Latino father when Lisa was a child. Her childhood was difficult and characteristically unstable. She recalled instances of physical abuse from her alcoholic father starting when she was three years old, "He lived off welfare and drink."

> Well, we had bunk beds. I remember he came in and picked me up by my shoulders and threw me down on the floor. That's all I remember. I don't remember anything else, and that's when I was three. I was very small.

Throughout her early childhood instances of physical abuse were followed by service interventions. Lisa described in detail how the problems she experienced in childhood set the stage for subsequent problems in her adolescence and young adulthood.

I was in and out of the hospital ten, fifteen, twenty times a year. I told my school about it, and my school intervened. They put me, my brother, and my sister in a foster home for a week, or two weeks, called us all liars, and sent us back home. I left, that's when I was nine. . . . When I was nine years old, my dad called my mom, my real mom, and said, "You know, I don't want her anymore." This was when they made me go home after the foster home, when I had run away. I went home to get some of my stuff, and my dad trapped me in the house and called my mom. My mom said, "Do you want to come and live with me?" and I said, "Yes." I had a way out. "Cool, you're in another state"; I was real excited about that. But I kept running away for awhile. For a couple of months, they kept putting me in foster homes, and I kept running away. Finally, they felt there was no alternative so they sent me to my mother. . . . Then she got involved with a Latin guy—my father's Latin—she got involved with a Latin guy and he was also a drinker. I thought, "Here we go again." Major flashback. I decided this was not for me, and I was getting in trouble all the time, being punished all the time for stuff I hadn't done. . . . My great aunt came down for a visit for a holiday and ended up taking me. So, I went to live on a farm. I stayed there. By that time I was so corrupt from being in a state home and being in foster homes and being on the run and being on the streets and using drugs, and drinking and smoking and doing this and doing that—by the time I went to the farm, there was no reform [laughs]. I was already a hellion. It was impossible for me to settle down. Because I was already used to moving about. So I ended up running away from there. That's when I started traveling.

She has "been traveling ever since." She claimed to have been in hundreds of foster homes, and learned to "be mature, be loud, get attention, and everybody takes care of you." Because of her unstable home life, she did not obtain a formal education.

I really only completed fifth grade. . . . I went to school. I'd go for three days to one school and then they'd put me in a new foster home. I'd go to another school and then I'd run away and I wouldn't be in school. Then I would come back, and I missed so much school that I couldn't keep up with my grade. The last time I ever attended school was ninth or tenth grade. I did my GED. That was it.

Lisa smoked marijuana and dropped acid during the periods she was living on the streets. After running away from the farm, she developed an appreciation for travel and learned how to use the social service system to her benefit.

I think when I left there, I called the police. I said I was a runaway and I wanted to go home. I was from the Northwest, so they couldn't force me to stay in that state because that's not where I was from. So they put me on an airplane, which I thought was the most exciting thing in the whole world. I'd never been on a plane before, and it was a free ride. I went back West on a plane. For some strange reason, I started running away out of state on purpose so that they would have to fly me back every time. I'd call and say, "Oh yes, I'm a runaway, and I'm tired of this state, so can you please send me home?" . . . They would buy me a plane trip ticket and put me on an airplane. Old men used to give me their little alcohol, and I used to get drunk on the way back. I would land and they'd put me in a lockup facility or another shelter home or another foster home.

Lisa claimed to have been in forty-eight states since age thirteen. She had consensual sex for the first time with a male at age fourteen while in a foster home, and she became pregnant. She became pregnant an additional three times before she turned twenty-four.

I found that being pregnant, you get a lot of attention. Being a young person, going through these programs or whatever. I used to like that. It didn't seem like reality because the baby wasn't big enough to be kicking, so it wasn't a reality to me. It was a game, a game of attention, a game of, "Oh, I'm pregnant, and a really important person." That's what I used it for. After I had the miscarriage, I really understood what was going on, and I went through a lot. Finally, I realized what was really happening. I mean it was real. It was a painful miscarriage. I started bleeding and everything was over with. I had the labor; I was sitting on the toilet. I was three months pregnant, and the baby was there in the toilet, and I'm looking at it. It doesn't bother me on a conscious level. On a subconscious level, it bothers me that I had a miscarriage and I wasn't taking care of myself. I could have. As far as the miscarriage, I never really dealt with it, or thought about it, or took time to think about it.

Shortly after her miscarriage, she ran away, lived on the street again, and began to snort crank. Her living situation alternated between foster care and homelessness.

I was on the street more than I was in foster homes. I would have five to ten placements a month, in foster care, but I would run away all the time. In between foster homes, I would be on the street. . . . From the age of fourteen to seventeen that's all I did was travel, and come back, and travel and come back—foster homes, group homes, streets, drugs, everything. I ended up pregnant again when I was seventeen. . . . I found out I was pregnant, and I was using at the time a lot of crank. I was at the point where I was real tired of doing crank. I was getting bored being high, so I was quitting anyway. It was a good excuse to quit, so I quit using crank and drugs. I was very healthy. I didn't drink; I barely smoked when I was pregnant. I was in a foster home. I guess I had been there a month. I was working at the same time. I was trying to save money to move out on my own or find out what I was going to do. Because I was in a foster home, and I was becoming an adult, having a baby so I had to figure out what to do. I was working in a fast food restaurant and I'd come home, and the foster home would refuse to feed me dinner at night because I had missed it because I was working. I was getting really sick. I wasn't getting nutritious food; I wasn't getting three meals a day. I wasn't getting what I needed, when I needed it. They had put me on probation for being a runaway. I had an officer and I called her and I said, look this foster home is not giving me adequate this, adequate that, this is what is happening with me, this is no good for me. Put me back into the juvenile home I was in. I begged her. I said, "Put me in there, please. You've got to put me in there until I have this baby. I can be healthy and gain weight there." She says, "No, no, I can't do that because you request it." I said, "Okay, fine. What will it take for you to put me back in there?" She thought I was kidding, so she said, "Well, take off out of state, and that will get you back there." I said, "Okay, I'll call you from somewhere; I'll call you in about a week." So, I took off; here, I'm pregnant and I'm pretty sick you know, and I went out of state and I called her up. I said, "Well, I think I did it. I'm out of state, and I'm really sick, and you've got to help me." So she sent me a plane ticket and they brought me back there, and they put me back into the facility I wanted. I'm glad they did, because that was the only place that I was going to be healthy, get the food I needed, gain weight, and get twenty-four-hour prenatal care. I went straight from there to the hospital. I was in the hospital about a week. After that week, they sent me back to the Northwest. That's when the HIV test thing happened. They did an HIV test on my blood without my permission.

Lisa and her newborn daughter were returned to the Northwest and placed in a "broken-down motel." Her social service worker visited them a week later to discuss the baby's HIV status.

She came over and said, "I have to tell you something." She told me that my daughter tested positive for HIV. She was asleep, so I broke out crying. It lasted for five minutes, and I snapped out of it. My life got back together. I got back to being a mother and I didn't think about it twice. After I left the motel, they put me in a foster home with a woman who considered herself an honorable citizen, someone who helped others. She took me and my daughter in, and we got real close. I never had like a real mom, so we got real close. She knew exactly what to do to get close to me. To make a long story short, what she wanted from me was my daughter. Because she saw that she could make money off my daughter easy and that's what she was after. . . . My daughter was an HIV-positive baby; she started a million dollar program for my baby. . . . I didn't see it coming. I had no idea what was going on. She'd pay for an apartment for me, and furnish it, and help me get my life together. She'd take care of my daughter for me until I was ready to get her back; then she'd give her back to me. It seemed like a good idea. I thought my daughter will be well taken care of until I can take care of her. When I moved out, she called social services and told them that I abandoned my daughter there, and that I didn't want her anymore. Automatically, I was in the system; I had been in the system all my life. Automatically, I was this bad person. I didn't want my child. I treated my child like a dog, and I never took care of her. . . . They got attorneys and case workers and battles were fought. It lasted for about a year. After a year, I couldn't take it anymore so I signed adoption papers for my daughter. I had no idea what I was doing at the time, but I did it, that's all. I was seventeen. . . . After the adoption papers went through, this woman published an article about my daughter. The title was "My Miracle Baby"; her miracle baby! She was this godsend that helped out this poor little child [Lisa]. This poor little child [Lisa] who had a child used to feed her baby alcohol. All these things that weren't true: that I was a drug addict, and I chose drugs and the streets over my child. . . . all kinds of things in a public paper. It was on the front page of the Sunday paper. I was really devastated, I didn't know what to do. I lived my life in a numb fashion, for a long time. Then I got pregnant with my son, and it was like "Cool. I can do it this time, because I know what not to do this time."

Lisa believed she was infected with HIV when she was thirteen years old and lived on the streets.

When I was thirteen, I was tied to a bed, and I had drugs intravenously put into my arm. I know that's when I got it because I never shot drugs, and I just know that's where I got it. . . . He was a very filthy, nasty, sick man. That's where I got it; he took me into a motel and tied me down.

The only reason Lisa ever had consensual sex with men was to "get kids." She never informed the fathers of her children of her pregnancy nor of their paternity. She wanted it that way.

We simply went in the bedroom, we fucked, got it over with, and that was it. I didn't know them. They didn't know me either–that was it. . . . I've had relationships with women. I've had sex with men.

During and after her second pregnancy, Lisa had four stable relationships with women and a handful of brief lesbian sexual encounters. Her gay consciousness originally developed when she was on the streets.

Gay was no big deal; on the street, everybody was going to be bi or gay–nobody cared. I just grew into it. Someone took me to one of the underage clubs and it was a gay club and I had no idea what it was. I mean I knew what it was. Because even when I was a kid, I always used to look at my sister. I could never figure out why I was so intrigued by my sister. When I saw women kissing, I thought, "Oh." I kind of choked up there for a minute, and then I thought, "Oh well, this is cool." That's how I was broken into it, and that's when I was fourteen.

Lisa had brief sexual affairs with women from then on. She was seventeen and living on her own when she met twenty-three-year-old Janet, her first "real relationship," at a lesbian club in the Northwest. She told Janet about her HIV status on their first date. Lisa was self-conscious about her HIV infection and her attractiveness to others as a result.

It was the first date I had with her, I told her. After that, I'm like, "Oh, you don't want to be with me; you don't want to ruin your life." While I'm saying this she's looking at me and she says, "Well, you let me be the judge of that; that's my decision not yours, thank you very much. I have decided to keep with you if you don't have any problem with that." I shut up real quick and it ended up being a real warm relationship. We ended up being together for a year and a half.

Lisa and Janet lived with Janet's parents. Later they moved into an apartment together, and their "lives went to hell." According to Lisa, Janet's parents thought that she had "turned" Janet gay.

They knew she was gay before me. But they just thought it was a phase, and they didn't like any part of that phase. I was a part of that phase.

Their relationship ended when Lisa, then working the graveyard shift, discovered Janet was having sex with another woman. It was a year later before Lisa began another relationship with twenty-five-year-old Becky, whom she met at the same lesbian nightclub. Their relationship, which Lisa described as sexually exciting and fulfilling, involved weekend crack and alcohol usage, and was characterized by frequent arguments. They seemed to have little in common except an intense mutual sexual attraction. The relationship ended after six months, and Lisa immediately wanted to get pregnant. After becoming pregnant for the third time, she began a six-month relationship with another woman. At first the woman was supportive of the pregnancy.

She loved it; well, she liked it. She liked the idea, but she was nervous. She never was interested in anything like that, and knowing that I was HIV also, at that time tripped her out. . . . It was a tough subject for a while. Then it got to the point where she wanted to bow out; she wasn't ready for something like that, so she went about her business and I went about mine. . . . It bothered me, but nothing was going to get in my way, not even a woman. I was going to have this child.

Three months later at age twenty and after her third pregnancy, Lisa had her second child, a son. He did not seroconvert HIV positive, but nevertheless was soon taken away from Lisa. Again despondent and alone, she left the Northwest and traveled, staying for extended periods in the Southwest. Social service workers would provide her with the names and contacts of providers in other cities, and she was able to obtain assistance shortly after arrival in different places. In 1991, she came to California and became a client of The Program, which by that time was a prominent community-based agency for youth living with HIV and AIDS. A service provider in the Southwest telephoned the director of The Program, and arrangements were made for Lisa before she arrived. The Program provided housing, support, and counseling services, which for the most part she avoided. She was the only female in The Program, and she had problems adjusting to the other clients, who were predominantly young gay men.

> You have to listen to gay men go on and on and on at the mouth. Street talk–I get tired of street talk, nasty-mouthed street talk. . . . I avoided them [the other clients] for the most part. I didn't sit and have intelligent conversations with any of them. Some of them don't seem like they have enough upstairs [points to her head] because they've used so many drugs for so long. They're not conversational. So I don't put myself in that position.

She remained in The Program for four months before finding work as a truck driver and leaving California for a year and a half. After driving around the western United States, she lost her job and was stranded in Arizona. She knew she could obtain help back in California and returned. The first thing she did when she returned was call The Program.

> I called up and told them I was here. I told them the bind I was in, and it was handed to me. "Okay Lisa, don't worry about it; take a cab over here." I had no bus fare. I was in a lot of trouble; the bank wouldn't cash my check. I was in a real bad situation. I didn't know where I was going to stay, all these things, and boom! They paid for my cab fare, they brought me down and they got me into a hotel as long as I wanted it.

Her Program-assigned caseworker paid for a hotel room for Lisa that was located on the same block of buildings that housed The Program. She was provided with a one-room studio, without television or telephone. She appeared isolated, lonely, and alone even though The Program was nearby. In her words she was "angry, not isolated." After being away from The Program for over a year, she returned and was the only female. She continued to have a difficult time relating to the young gay men in The Program–Damian, Jordan, Ethan, Mark, and Jared, all of whom were still heavily involved in street life, including substance use and sex work. Even though she had similar life experiences, Lisa described herself as different from them.

Because I'm tired. I've already experienced a lot of things. I have no further wishes to experience much of anything else. I've grown up and gotten wiser; it's taught me a lot. Most people are still immature and not facing what they need to face. They're HIV; they're whatever it is in their lives; they need to face it. They don't care, they use drugs, and it's a bunch of street garbage. . . . They choose to act like they're five years old; they act like they're twelve years old; they act like they're fifteen years old. After a while, it becomes a habit. It's not something they will give up; it becomes the way you talk, the way you present yourself, the way you come across. It's a habit. After a while, you've done it for so long, you don't even realize you do it. These are hard people to deal with.

Lisa, in contrast to other youth in The Program, had gone to other HIV-related agencies for support and counseling. She wanted to meet others who had experiences similar to hers. As a long-term client, she knew how to use the system. According to Lisa she was "very good at acquiring information" and had been her whole life. She specifically tried to find other lesbians who were living with HIV. However, her experiences in individual and group activities did not meet her expectations or needs. She described this dilemma in detail.

When I first started going to these women's groups that were HIV-positive women's groups, or groups specifically for HIV or AIDS people, all I listened to was "Poor me, oh my God, I'm dying of this," or "Oh my God, I caught this yesterday," or "Oh my God, I'm on this new medication." Forget all you people. I don't want to sit and talk about how you are dying and how sick you are. That's fine once in a while, but to sit and analyze it and analyze it and analyze it, and tear it apart, the conversation gets old. I don't want to sit and listen to people that are dying and complaining and moaning and groaning and sitting in their own mess. I don't want to hear it. I don't have time for that! That's why I don't go to groups; I don't have time for that. . . . There is little talk about what somebody did that day to help themselves; they don't talk about those things. All everybody talked about in the women's group–

everybody in there was straight; there was not one lesbian women but myself—all I heard was, "I had some sex last week," or "Oh, I didn't have any this week," or "Oh, I'm being deprived," or "Oh, I met this new guy and I don't know how to tell him I'm HIV positive so I can get some." I don't want to hear that. I don't. I don't know what I wanted to hear or what I expected to hear, but those were not the things. . . . With gay men, the only thing on their mind is the next man, or "Oh God, I'm so sick." With straight women, it is sex this, sex that, "I'm horny. I want some. How do I get it?" I don't want to hear that either. But when it comes to lesbian women, that's not all they want to talk about. It's an automatic thing; they already have their own issues to talk about and it's about some immature thing like, "Oh, I'm dying." It's more serious. . . . I doubt that there are many women who are lesbian that are HIV positive. But those that are out there, have a desperate need. A lot of them are committing suicide, a lot of them are trying to kill themselves, and they're finding themselves in the same place I do, up against a wall. Because they have already tried the straight women's groups, and they don't work for them. They've tried the gay men's groups like I am now. I go to this all-gay-men group that does nothing for me. They're not like me. I can't associate with those people, I can't disassociate myself because I'm HIV positive, but I can't tell them my problems. Nobody understands, nobody. They can't relate, there's just no relation, and with straight women there's no relation.

After living for six months in the transient hotel near The Program, Lisa moved into a long-term residential hotel in the downtown area. She obtained a radio, television, and telephone. She started to feel more comfortable about her living situation. Nevertheless, she wanted to find an apartment away from all the drugs and sex work. She felt she would bide her time and look for a better place. Lisa forced herself to go to one of the few lesbian bars in the area, and she hoped to find another lover. She also wanted to have another baby. She placed a personal telephone advertisement in a local newspaper and dated fifteen women who responded, "Not dating them as lovers, but trying just to go out and have fun as friends." She specified in her ad that she preferred policewomen and firefighters, "those in uniform." She dated a number of both. She emphasized that she liked the uniform, but even more "the control behind the uniform." Although her advertisement specified that she was looking for women, more than ten men responded. She paraphrased the typical telephone calls of the men who responded to her advertisement.

> "I have this really nice penis and you'd really like it and I could change your world and you'd never want to be a lesbian again." All this little ego weird stuff they like to do. But, it doesn't change my world and it never would. It never could. I have no interest.

Not satisfied with the responses she got to her own advertisement, Lisa responded to Jill's. Jill, who eventually played an important role in Lisa's life, was a thirty-one-year-old medical receptionist, "a very big woman, not obese big, but big boned, muscled out." Lisa described what attracted her to Jill's advertisement.

> She was really old-fashioned. She's not into someone who is running around in the bar scene. It sounded like me. On our first real date, she came over to my place for coffee. After that, I went over to her house and I ended up spending the night. I told her I was HIV positive, and we talked about it. It was really hard for her at first. . . . And we had excellent sex; we had excellent sex!

Lisa starting spending most of her time at Jill's house. She met Jill's parents, and she and Jill discussed moving in together. The relationship intensified. They discussed "marriage."

> Too fast. She just signed a lease on this apartment for another year, I think for a full year. She asked me to marry her. She said, "Well, at the end of my lease, you're going to marry me. We're going to go to Mexico and get married." She's going on and on and on. I said, "This sounds wonderful," and she got real explicit, saying "I'll buy you roses and this is the hotel we

will be in, and this is how much it is going to cost, and this is going to be what we'll do all night long." Planned to the T, right? She even started looking at two-bedroom apartments.

Lisa wanted to work in the medical field, and the more time she spent with Jill, the more jealous and angry she became hearing Jill talk about her work in a hospital. Jill complained about Lisa's laziness, and told her "get yourself on the phone, find a school, and go now!" Lisa recalled how Jill forced her into action.

> She says, "Well, if your going to be around me and you have a dream, you'll have to go for it. Because I'm not quitting my job because you can't stand it, and it's killing you because you want to do it."

Lisa enrolled in a medical assistant program at a technical school. The Program paid her application fee and bought her nursing uniform and stethoscope. She was excited about the course her life was taking. However, soon after starting school, she learned she was pregnant again, and less-positive aspects of Jill's character became more evident.

> One night she got really upset. We got into an argument. She really wanted to know something important about me. She asked about my kids, because I told her I had kids. I finally broke down and cried and told her the whole story of why and how and where and when and who and what and all. I was real upset. It really was an emotional night. The conversation was about appreciating me for who I am. Not letting HIV get in the way or anything like that. I have this problem: I say things that I'm thinking without thinking about the consequences of what I'm saying before I say it. I made a comment that I didn't want someone feeling sorry for me. And I guess the way I said it, she thought I was feeling sorry for myself and I was shutting her out of my life and my mind and my thoughts. She got really upset, I mean really upset. I assumed that she was masturbating in the other room. Here I was emotional and everything, and I thought all she was thinking about was sex. I find out she was crying; I mean, she was upset too. . . . . She's a real sexual

person, and when she gets stressed out, she becomes, you know, sexual. I got real upset; I had a right to be upset. If that's what she was doing, here I am being all emotional, and she gets me to break down, and she goes in and masturbates. It's like I'm not good for sex. I'm not good enough for her. What am I doing here? So I got real upset about it. I kept making comments. I can't remember what they were, but they really upset her. She didn't hit me, but she got real physical for a minute. I said to myself, "How does life look?" I said, "Check yourself; this is it." I said, "I've had a dad like this; he taught me very well. I'm over it right now—this is it." That was it. I found out she ended up going to a therapist the next day. She called in sick at work and went to a therapist. If I were to say, "I'm not going to stay with you because of your anger and because you could get physical with me," it would be the same thing as her saying to me I'm not going to stay with you because you're HIV positive and you need to work on that. It's a double-edged sword.

Given her history of physical abuse, Lisa wanted to be cautious with Jill. However, valuing the strong sexual attraction between them, Lisa made concessions and remained in the relationship.

It makes me feel really good. Because she tells me how our sex life is really good and stuff. That makes me feel good. It's like, God, I would hate to lose a lover because my sex isn't perfect, you know? She's constantly saying that she loves making love with me. She always talks about how I look, my nails, all these things—it's always appearance. When it comes to how she feels about me, I don't hear much. But yet, the HIV conversations she puts her heart into. She wants to talk about it. She brings it up. It makes me feel good. This woman really wants to know, and this woman is really interested in me. It can't be just sex, to put all her time and energy into these conversations. She's a really blunt person and she will ask me bluntly, like I realized that I still have breast milk. I've had two kids and they're both older now, but I still have breast milk. If someone's sucking on my breast then it just automatically starts producing breast milk. Because I have ducts that have been triggered by having kids. The other day she wound up getting a little milk out of my breasts. She says "Babies get it from milk." She flipped out, "right?" I said, "Okay, wait a minute." I said, "Jill, you are correct, that is how babies can get it from their mothers. But, you're an adult, okay, and there's a certain amount of HIV that's going to be in the milk. You don't thrive and live off my breasts twenty-four hours a day. There's a big difference. You could swallow a tablespoon and it's not going to jump inside your blood cells and start attacking you. It's not." I breast-fed my kids, knowing I was HIV positive, and my son didn't become positive. He's not positive to this day. I only say what I know, and I have been through it.

Similar to seromixed gay male couples in which only one partner is HIV positive, lesbian couples often take precautions during sexual activities. According to Lisa, her HIV status was always a concern for the couple.

It was a scary thing for me, because she says for me to keep it in my mind that she's negative and I'm positive, and that I have to understand. And I tell her I do understand, but you also have to give me the same understanding. I do have it, and what I go through and how it affects me when you bring this up. We talk about it a lot. And this is the first lover I've had where we talk about it quite a bit. If she has a question, I know she'll ask me. If there's a problem, she'll say it. We use gloves; we have safe sex. We practice different things at different times. I like it because the relationship I had before with my ex-lover it never came up! It bothered me and made me feel like she didn't care. I mean, if you can't care about a part of me, then you can't care about me. I'm realizing that a way that someone shows me they care about me is to bring it up. Tell me what they think, or talk about it because you feel like you need to talk about it, or it's an issue, or it bothers you. It's something. Although it makes me feel uncomfortable, I enjoy knowing that she has concerns for herself and for me—not just a totally one-sided thing.

Lisa and Jill used gloves during sexual activity, both as a precautionary measure and also as part of their sex play.

> It's actually funny because it works out really well. She'll get this sexual streak. She'll go to the bathroom and on her way back she'll grab one glove for each of us and stick them in her pocket. It's like okay, if it comes up. . . . She wears gloves because she has a skin disorder, dry skin and stuff, so she has cracks in her fingers all the time. . . . I think she likes me to use gloves because I have long nails. . . . She sticks them under the pillow before we go to bed; it's really cute. I mean she'll stick one under each pillow before we go to bed, so at night if something comes up, its right there.

Their communication regarding sexuality was more direct and meaningful than with previous lovers. They explored their sexuality more freely. Even though she had experienced physical abuse with men, Lisa enjoyed rough sexual activities with Jill.

> I like having my arms held down sometimes. I like for her to get really rough with me, like control me sexually. But not so rough that I'm going to get all bruised up, not really a big major S&M thing. To know that someone's there with the muscle control. I like that, and she's always liked doing that to somebody. We had a big conversation about that, and that's what draws both of us to each other. We allow each other further sexual exploration than our past lovers did. It's been a really good experience, a nice experience. . . . One time she started to hold my arms down and I tried to move them and I said, "Oh, hold them down again," and just from there, she knew then, no problem. . . . We talk about what would please us. We do everything. It's like, "What do you want me to do to you?" or, "How do you want it done?" or, "What would make you feel good?" I said, "I don't want to make love to you rough; I want to make love to you nice and soft, and emotional." It was the neatest thing, because we realized that we could do both. We could be really sentimental, and we could also still be sexual in ways that are fantasy.

After six months, busy with school and pregnant for the forth time, Lisa ended the relationship with Jill. Jill could not accept Lisa's pregnancy. Lisa, finding condoms around Jill's house, suspected she was having sex with men. The rough sex that had been at times enjoyable became augmented with physical abuse outside of the bedroom and came to resemble Lisa's past experiences with men. Angry and hurt, Lisa refocused on her pregnancy and school, "No woman, no animal, no man, no human, no God, no anything on this earth will affect my school, but me." She continued to receive assistance from The Program while she attended classes. She kept her HIV status from everybody at school. She refused to participate in class-related blood drawing exercises, claiming she was a hemophiliac. After three months in school, Lisa was in an automobile accident. She was hospitalized with a broken leg, and dropped out of school. Still living in a downtown hotel, "a stressful place to be," she stayed home most of the time preparing for the birth of her baby.

> Where I live, if I come out, there are drug addicts every-where. There are whores everywhere. I am sick to death of having it in my face. When I go to The Program, that's all I see, and I can't deal with it. . . . I don't want to have street people in my life at this point. I don't care to have HIV in my life, I don't care to have drug addicts in my life, I don't care to have prostitutes in my life, and I don't want them around my child. Not that I'm better than anybody else. That has nothing to do with it. The fact is that I left that in my past and I want it to stay there. The more you're around those people, the more you'll find friends like them, and I'm tired of them.

Lisa only left her hotel room to eat at The Program ("to make my food last longer at home"), obtain prenatal care, or pick up the baby furniture and clothes donated by various youth or maternal social service programs ("to ensure the baby is not taken away"). From the beginning, Lisa insisted on having a female obstetrician, "The reason why is because I hate men and I choose a female doctor because I'm gay. That's it in a nutshell." She refused to speak about HIV when she sought prenatal care, and refused to take any exper-imental drugs.

The first day I went in I said, "I don't want to hear anything about AIDS. I don't want to hear nothing about HIV, or that's HIV related because that's not true and if it is I'll know it. I don't need you to tell me that," and I said "That's the end of this conversation. I do not wish to speak about this topic any further throughout my whole pregnancy." That was it. If I hadn't said that, I know how it works. I've done this for many, many years! I know how it works, every little sniffle you get, Oh, HIV this, HIV that, "Let me give you some drugs; get on AZT." I'm not into this experimental crowd. I am me. If I'm going to die, let me die. . . . Thank you for the information, thank you for trying to be supportive, but I don't want to hear this. I am sick to death of people trying to convince me to take drugs. It's pissing me off actually. It's making me very angry.

Lisa attempted to control how providers dealt with her, setting the conditions and parameters of the relationships. Throughout her lover relationships, pregnancies, and travels, Lisa maintained monthly contact with service providers in many cities and states. Some of these relationships extended back twelve years, and constituted a pseudo-family for her. She had little contact with her mother, sister, and brother; they only wanted to talk about a past she was trying to forget. Dependent upon the social service system for over half her life, first as a abused child, then as a runaway youth, next as a youth living with HIV, and most recently, as a young pregnant mother with HIV, Lisa knew how to use the system to her advantage.

I'm not going to lie. I have tried to *use the system to my advantage*, mainly because of fatigue. Not to my advantage where everything I say is 100 percent a lie, but sometimes it takes some exaggeration to get disability, and it takes a lot. I've seen a doctor for those particular reasons. As far as being sick and all that, no, I have never had any HIV problems. But any little thing that happens to me they assume is HIV. So I let them assume that, and I go, "Okay, sure, no problem, fine."

After everything she had been through in her twenty-four years, she remained optimistic and ready to act on whatever opportunities arose.

I want to stay home for the first year of the baby's life, but I still want to further my career in the medical field. I don't know how soon to do that. I don't know if I should go back to school. I don't have an answer for that. God, I wish I did. Because I'm nervous as hell. I mean I have options, but I'm not sure which I'm going to take.

During her pregnancy, research was publicized that indicated mothers who use AZT during pregnancy had a better chance of delivering HIV negative babies (25 percent chance dropped down to 8 percent if on AZT). She agreed to use AZT, and had a healthy, HIV-negative baby in early 1994.

When Lisa turned twenty-four, The Program needed to transition her to adult services. They concluded that she needed to be in a program, with twenty-four-hour supervision. They placed her in a residential program, one for HIV-positive mothers with babies. Lisa was successful in the new program for a short time. However, according to her primary service provider, in the summer of 1994, she reverted to old patterns, packed her few possessions, and left with the baby.

She was being obstinate about care of the baby and not listening to people. She breast-fed the baby for about a day, and we worked with her around that. She brought it up and we moved in on it. We said, "You can't do that, you know that. If you do that, we'll get Child Protective Services involved. We are going to move on it." She backed off, and said she would listen. You're dealing with a triple-diagnosis kid, with mental health issues, besides the other issues she had. That's when we really put the pressure on her to get her into a program, which we did. We said to her, "You know you're twenty-four, you need to be in this program. If you leave this program, we will not house you." She wasn't thrilled about it; she's discharged from our program. She eventually left the adult residential mother's program and went East. Nobody has heard from her since. She bolted from the program, took the baby, and went East. We don't even know where she is. It's totally predictable. Really since before 1987, before HIV became part of her life, that was the way she functioned. Her total pattern was to do okay for awhile, and then she would destabilize. That is her whole pattern; she has no internal locus of control. It was one thing when she was alone, but now she has the baby. She destabilizes so rapidly and where does that leave the baby? She ends up with males or females who are destructive, abusive, that was her pattern. She was a classic borderline. That's the way she survives. . . . I don't see her keeping this baby either.

Chapter 10

"My Track Record": Mark

*It was then the fashion, as it has been at almost all
times and places, to be stupid, mean, and more vile
than one could have believed; he was vile, mean,
and stupid, more than others because of the circles
into which his beauty threw him.*

–Paul Verlaine, *Charles Husson* (In Cory, 1953)

*I ask myself if in the days of antiquity
glorious Alexandria possessed a more superb-looking youth,
a lad more perfect than he–who had been wasted:
Of course no statue or painting was ever done of him . . . .
and by common debauchery, so wretched, he was destroyed.*

–C.P. Cavafy, *Days of 1909, 1910, 1911* (In Dalven, 1961)

Mark was a twenty-year-old, gay-identified, white male who was periodically homeless for six years. He was of medium height, of slight build, with bushy auburn hair. He frequently wore jeans, a "Psycho University" sweatshirt, and well-worn graffiti-covered athletic shoes. He was animated and spoke in a rapid, sarcastic manner. His attention span varied based upon the amount of speed he used. He reeked of cigarettes, and he sometimes exuded a toxic, chemical body odor. He was very bright and witty, if not "catty" in how he described his life and others. Mark was a native of California and was raised by his grandparents. His mother and father gave him up for adoption when he was a small child. Both parents had histories of alcohol and drug abuse.

Like Lisa, Mark was a well-known "veteran" among the service bureaucracy, and he had more knowledge about the social service system than many long-term providers. He was genuinely proud of his "records" for length and amount of placements at youth shelters over the years, and the number of "squats" he had lived in. He believed he was given more opportunities than other youths in his predicament because service providers "liked him better than others." Mark was actively involved in sexual activity for money or goods since age thirteen. He was dependent upon social agencies for food vouchers, General Assistance, and housing. He was a long-term client of The Program. He participated in Program-sponsored activities on a daily basis with the other "tweakers" (methamphetamine users) or "cereal-holics" (those who eat Captain Crunch and Fruity Pebbles). Mentally, they all escaped through daily communal viewing of *Star Trek: The Next Generation* at The Program. He knew Ethan and Jared well, and had met Lisa. In general, he did not befriend or socialize with others away from The Program. He used varying amounts of speed routinely. He was usually "running speed" or "coming down" while participating in Program activities. As is common with most long-term speed users, he had learned to manage his chronic drug use. Mark seldom reflected on his drug-dependent lifestyle and HIV status, and believed that concentrating on these aspects of his life only accelerated the onset of clinical symptoms of AIDS. He took life on a day-to-day and a high-to-high basis, and his long-term expectations were few. For example, he did not plan to obtain his GED because he did not expect to reap the benefits of any effort he might put forth. He was content to go to the Program's support group twice a week, shoot-up alone or with his two or three friends, and work the infrequent "trick." He had little contact with his grandparents, and his social network was limited to those involved in the sex and drug world he knew for over six years. In remembering the street scene of his adolescence, Mark named many former friends, johns, and street regulars who had died of AIDS. However, his own HIV status had not affected his behavior or lifestyle. Although, he had "burned out" of the daily grind of being a street sex worker, he believed this would have happened whether he had been infected or not. As he emphasized, "that life gets old after a while, and anyway, there's always someone prettier coming along."

Mark was 13 when he first arrived in Northern California, and soon learned that he could earn money through full-time sexual activity for money on the streets or in gay-oriented bars. He liked the attention he received that had been lacking in his previous family and peer relationships. He remembered being high the first time that he had sex with another male, an adult, when he was thirteen years old. Marijuana made the "whole sexual thing" easier. In subsequent years, he experimented with crack cocaine and heroin and had a long stretch of alcohol abuse that "clouded over" his life for five years. In fact, during interviews, he had a hard time remembering specific activities during this period. He did remember clearly that he began speed use in pill form at age sixteen and had "shot up" (run) on an almost daily basis since age seventeen. His first inject-able speed experience was with an older man with whom he lived for a short period of time. He remembered this older man "shooting him" up in the forearm during a sexual episode. At that time he believed he was in love. He did not have similar "fantasies" afterward.

For seven years his housing situation varied and was unstable, reflecting the general lack of affordable or safe housing for home-less youth. Initially, he stayed for eight months in a squat, "I lived in squats a lot. You go there to sleep. You go there to sleep, wake up, and leave." He would shower at the public aquatic center. Short-term and extended stays followed in youth shelters, and with older men who would "keep" him for extended periods of time during his middle adolescence. He was unable to identify the exact incident that led to his HIV infection, as he was involved in many risk activities for so long. He tested HIV positive at age sixteen. At that time he was using drugs, experiencing psychological problems, and was suicidal. The Program medical staff decided not to tell him that he was HIV infected at the time, deciding to wait until he was stabilized and could deal with the results of his test. He was origi-nally told that he tested HIV negative.

They were probably right. But still it's not their place. They shouldn't have lied and said it was negative. They should have said that my results weren't back yet, or taken another test or something—not directly lied, and said "Oh yes, it came back negative." So, I'm thinking "Great, it's negative. I'll fuck who I want, and I'll shoot dope with who I want."

A week later during a seven-day speed run, Mark was hospitalized by the police on a "5150" or danger to self or others. He slept in the hospital for four days without waking, and was discharged with the knowledge that he had tested HIV positive.

Since late 1993, Mark has lived alone in a downtown "skid row" hotel room provided by The Program. He had no kitchen facilities or television, he listened to the radio when he was home while running speed. He religiously checked his horoscope in the daily paper. The rest of the day he was out obtaining money for speed "shopping sprees." He did not socialize with others at the hotel (other drug users and sex workers), and his immediate primary social world was composed of his "speed supplier" and the "johns" he still knew from the streets. He did not remember the first time he had sex for money.

> I don't even remember. I really have done too much dope. I just don't remember that. The first date I ever pulled. I've pulled a lot of dates [laughs]; I have a wide base. . . . I pulled a lot of dates with people I already knew that I saw again and again and again. . . . I've made my fair share.

For Mark the interconnection between drug use and sexual activity was direct, and while high-risk sexual activity may not have necessarily resulted, the psychologically numbing effects that drugs had on his sexual activity were manifest in the following illustration. This episode also illustrates the financial benefits sex work provided Mark, who refered to one particular john alternatively as "she" and "he."

> Like the big fat guy that picked me up one time, a long time ago, gave me three hundred dollars. She wasn't the most attractive thing in the world. Well, she says, "I'll give you three hundred dollars–one hundred dollars an hour." I had an hour to get to her house, right, and as soon as we got to her house, she gave me a hundred dollars. That's for the hour. An hour at her house, of which, thirty minutes of it I spent watch-

ing her television [laughs]. All she wanted to do—mind you, she's three hundred and seventy-something pounds—all she wanted to do was lay on top of me, and do nothing, but lay on top of me, because that's how she gets off, by laying on top of me. So I said, "For three hundred dollars, sure." He's hollering, "Okay?"—"Sure, I'm fine!" She gave me another hundred, and we got into the car and we came back to my room. When we got back she gave me another hundred. She wasn't attractive. If I wouldn't have been high on something, I never would have went with her [laughs].

When asked about his friends, Mark identified Daniel as the person he went to when he needed help. Daniel was his thirty-four-year-old "former lover," one of the main downtown drug suppliers. He provided Mark with a $20 bag of speed for free each day, and did not make sexual or financial demands in return. According to Mark, "He loves me."

> Never had sex with her. She was my husband. I don't have sex with my husband. I do his dope and I spend his money, but I don't have sex with her.

Mark twitched as he spoke. In general, he was lucid and forthcoming in discussing his life. He was very sensitive, if not overly self-critical. During all interviews he was usually high on speed and began the interviews in an affected speech pattern, which included references to "he" as "she," reflective of his socialization into the vernacular of the homosexual street scene. Since 1993 he had not actively been involved in full-time sexual activity for money although he did sometimes run into old johns and fell "into old patterns." From 1992 to 1994, he occasionally walked down the main hustling street ("my daily stroll") while high. If a car stopped, he did not say no to "advances." Even after such long-term drug use, he maintained a self-controlled manner and still distinguished potential risk situations while high.

> Oh yeah, she takes me, in this taxi, all the way up to the frickin' outside of town. The whole time she's sitting there, she's freebasing coke. I did maybe two hits and then I said,

"No, that's okay. I don't do that shit; I don't want any more."
She kept saying, this we, we, we, so I'm thinking okay, she's
talking, we, him, me, us, we. She's got this lover or something
that's upstairs, that she picked me up to come and mate with. I
said, "Oh no, wait a minute." I said, "No, no. I did not come
here to trick with your troll that's locked up in the attic." She
said well, blah-blah-blah. I said, "You know what? I just cannot be bothered. You got the wrong hooker." She said, "Well,
I thought you were working." I said that I was not working,
you chased me up the street, if I remember right [laughs]. If her
lover wants to pick me up, then her lover needs to get into a
taxi and drive over and pick me up for himself. Because who's
to say if I would have even gone with her lover.

Mark spent money easily, and took taxis whenever possible.
Through sex work or other illegal money-making activities, he had
episodic but continual contact with law enforcement officers. In
1993, Mark made additional money through "plastic scams,"
wherein he used stolen credit cards or worked "bank scams" and
forged signatures on checks. As a result he stopped frequenting the
streets, but not because of any fear of the police.

I found out that when you start working checks and paper
and having money all the time, you really don't want to hang
out on the street. The street people turn into a bunch of tired
bitches that you don't want to be around. Because none of
them have money, and all they want to do is work you for what
you have.

Similar to other youth looking for ways to obtain money for drug
habits, Mark focused less on sexual activity for money and increasingly more on profitable activities such as stealing checks or money
orders that he and others obtained from accessible mailboxes ("the
paper group, the plastic, the people who work checks and things").
He described an episode that subsequently landed him in jail.

So I took this check, which was good. I forget where it was
from, and it was for over three grand. So the check was good,
and I opened a bank account with the check in my name. And

we waited a couple of days for the check to clear, and it was a holiday weekend so I had to wait until Tuesday. . . . On Tuesday, I went to the bank and took out a hundred. On Wednesday, I went to the bank and deposited another check for about nine hundred and took out about fifteen hundred in cash, which we had split three ways with two other people. We did the same thing the next day, and took fifteen hundred out in cash and went shopping.

Mark spent the majority of this money on drugs, clothing, and a male "friend." His explanation of what happened next illustrates his frequent generosity, the central role drugs play, and concurrently the tenuous nature and lack of reciprocity in his relationships.

I got her extremely full [drugs]. I bought her dinner; I bought her brand new clothes; I gave her money for cigarettes and what have you. Then when she was leaving, she asked me for twenty dollars to pay her rent, and I said, "No." She had the nerve to sit there and read me because I wouldn't give her twenty dollars to pay her rent, after I gave her at least sixty dollars worth of dope without even thinking of getting anything in return. . . . I was inventorying all the things I did for her that day. . . . I'm like, "Wait a minute. What about the heroin I bought you?" I don't do heroin; I bought it for her. I took her out to lunch; I bought her a brand new outfit; it cost me over a hundred and fifty dollars. Plus, I gave her the money for the cigarettes. . . . "Wait a minute bitch, how many times did you come down and pay my rent? Please!" So she's not my friend anymore. She's tired.

Mark was eventually arrested trying to cash a stolen check at a bank. He was taken to the county jail, where he had been many times before. He described the experience in detail, including how young gay men were treated, as well as those living with HIV or AIDS.

They pulled up my warrant. I made a report; I made a statement, and I did all the stupid stuff they make you do. You go to jail and get processed. You sit there for hours, and then you go in and you get countless fingerprints done. You sit there for hours and hours and wait to go in the back. I could not wait to get to where all the fags were. Everyone that I'd been looking for all weekend was sitting there, the gay tank [laughs]. I knew just about everybody. That's where all the people from the street who get arrested go; everybody who runs through the street now and then. It is a very small city, and people who tweak are interconnected. Everybody who tweaks meets everybody else at some point in time. They run, they're at a dope dealer's house, and there are a couple of people there, and you meet tweakers. Most of us are HIV positive. . . . When you go to jail, they ask, "Do you have any illnesses we should know about, and have you been tested for TB?" They already knew that I had HIV from the several times I've been in jail. They had it in their computers. They say, "Okay, you have it; great, you get more food." You get more food because they think if you have HIV, you need to keep your weight up. They put you on a high-protein, high-calorie diet, which means you get more food. You have a life-threatening disease; they want to keep your health up. They don't want everybody in jail dying of AIDS. They want to keep you healthy.

The charges were dropped in twenty-four hours, and Mark was released from jail. Another "friend" who had a key to Mark's place believed Mark would be in jail for a long time and quickly sold all of Mark's possessions. Mark described him as "a tired, scandalous little bitch." Mark planned "to get even" with his former friend.

The bitch deserves it. I have not found her yet. Whatever anybody else does to her, that's somebody else getting her. On my behalf maybe, but they have other reasons for getting her, too. She's ripped them off, too. The bitch went into my house. I trusted her to give my keys and lock up my house. She went into my house and intentionally took all of my clothes, and then walked around the street bragging about it, saying, "Oh yeah, these are Miss Ma's clothes, I'm going to sell them.". . . It took me a long time to get all of those clothes, and now the only clothes that I have are the clothes that I'm wearing. They're all gone.

Disenfranchised, poor youths living with HIV often engaged in some form of illegal activity to support friends, lovers, and mostly their own drug habits. Many long-term substance users like Mark, found that speed was necessary to achieve sexual intimacy with strangers or potential lovers. Sexual activities for money provided cash to support drug habits and sometimes fleeting feelings of self-worth. These activities intensified during periods when personal sense of physical attractiveness was diminished due to feelings related to HIV and AIDS. For Mark, the constant use of methamphetamine also had negative social side effects including periods of self-imposed isolation.

> I mean, I was so tweaked out from the weekend that it wasn't even funny. I was in my room; I had my little friend, my little mouse. To this day, I don't even know if I actually saw a little mouse or not, but I thought I saw this little mouse. For a whole weekend, I was in my room and I'd pick up my coat, and I was trying to leave. I went like this [gestures] making sure there was no mouse in my coat. . . . I woke up Sunday morning and the first thing I did was puke out stomach acid. I said, "Gee, girl, when was the last time you ate?" [laughs]

Sexual activities were determined less by Mark's need for money than by his need for personal validation. In fact, he considered himself asexual. Sex for pleasure did not interest him anymore.

> I have to be on drugs to have sex with anybody, period. Because I do not enjoy having sex. I do not like to have sex. I do not go out and look for sex. I don't even masturbate. I don't do anything. I don't, like it's part of my manic depressiveness. Depressed people do not like to have sex. When they do, it's by themselves and it takes two minutes. I'm not interested in that. I have no use for it. That doesn't appeal to me. I won't unless I'm on speed.

Mark liked the fact that men still desired him. He distinguished between johns and tricks. Tricks were short-term sexual clients, whereas johns could be worked for long periods of time. If "worked right," they could be turned into "sugar daddies." He recalled encountering Tony, a sugar daddy he had worked for years.

He is in love with me. Another sorry son of a bitch who fell in love with me [laughs]. I said, "Well I want to buy some dope because I don't feel like featuring your cock today." She says, "Here's the money go buy the coke." . . . She likes to get people real full [high] and give them dope and have sex.

Like all of Mark's sexual partners, Tony was in his forties. Like Ethan, Mark emphasized that he was not attracted to men his own age who he believed were generally "stupid" and without direction. While he liked the stability he associated with older men (forties to fifties), he described them in general as dysfunctional, falling in "love too easily." Drug use, and speed use in particular, was a common feature of all of his relationships. Mark also acknowledged his own tendency to exploit others' desire to be close to him.

> *My track record*, I mean it's not exactly, you know, making the best time, the best mileage. I've left a lot of accidents on my highway of love [laughs]. I'd be the first person to tell you, "Excuse me, but you don't really want to be in love with me" [laughs]. Because I'll work you. If I know that somebody is going to do anything for me, I will work them. Not really bad, but I will work them. Like Daniel, Daniel came to pick me up in jail and gave me head. That's why she was the first person that I called. I knew he would pick me up, and I knew he would give me head.

Like Ethan, Mark depended on his former clients for assistance and support when he was stressed.

> He's not really a client anymore; we're more like friends. I call her at home when I'm stressed out. She lives out of town. She has a hot tub, her and her lover, a lovely house. When I get stressed out, I call her and say, "Come get me. I need to get out of town." And she comes and takes me. I go over to her house and watch her cable TV and sit in her hot tub. We don't do anything sexual, I just go over there. He comes here once in a while to meet me, or to buy dope.

An important condition for these relationships was the provision of drugs, and Mark was calculating in how he worked his "entourage."

> There is this group of people I call my entourage. Some people meet a lot of people and they rip them off. I don't. I keep the same four or five people, who were stupid enough to fall in love with me, and I work these same four or five people. Instead of ripping off a lot of people all the time, I keep the same five people, and I work them for months and months and months. If they want to come over, they have to give me a hit. It's not that I tell them that they have to give me a hit. It's understood that they're supposed to give me a hit.

The Program's service objectives for Mark were to promote his self-esteem, to provide him with realistic and achievable life alternatives and opportunities, and to develop his future orientation and "will to live." His self-description in one interview was telling.

> I'm a loner, not a group person. I always have been and I always will be.

Mark described his life as "running on autopilot." He did not feel he controlled his destiny but was resigned to his fate, which he believed was characteristically to "mess up." He described his unwillingness to change his life situation and patterns in a pessimistic way.

> Well, the reason I stay like this is because, as far as I can see, I'm going to die anyway. Why bother getting my shit together? I'll probably die before I do it [laughs]. . . . It's not the tea, to sit around wondering when I'm going to croak. Tomorrow, I could be in the hospital with tubes coming out of me.

Examples of speed use cessation among disenfranchised youth still engaged in street life were few (Rotheram-Borus et al., 1994). Mark modified his usage without any plans to totally quit. He developed the ability to function while high without major complications to his daily life. However, he remained in a social and developmental limbo, without plans for the future or legitimate employment possibilities. He relied on the assistance of service providers who had "taken care of him" for years. He received medical care every three months, and blood was drawn periodically for evaluation. The Program contracted a psychiatrist to see him on a regular basis, and the psychiatrist ordered medication for Mark's depression. He qualified to receive groceries from a AIDS food bank. Mark arranged for two bags to be delivered directly to his hotel room. He refused to wait in line at the food bank with others.

> I don't like having to go all the way down there. I don't like having to wait in line. I don't like having to deal with all those tired queens that look like they're dead. I don't like having to carry two bags of groceries all the way back. I'd rather just have them bring them to me. It's much easier, much simpler.

By late 1994, Mark received General Assistance and food stamps. He hoped to receive Social Security.

> I get one hundred and ten dollars worth of food stamps every month. I don't buy very much food with them, because I don't have anything to cook with. I might buy a loaf of bread and peanut butter and jelly and some KoolAid. With the rest of the stamps, I buy dope.

His high-risk sexual activity ceased years ago, and while his intravenous drug use continued, clean needles were more accessible. He claimed to be consistently bored. He smuggled a cat into his hotel room for company, and grew attached to her. He was eventually forced by the management to put her out. He had a telephone installed in his room. He spent a good amount of his time developing moneymaking scams. He placed an advertisement in the Personal Section in a gay newspaper. He established a telephone voice mailbox for responses.

> You record your own message. You leave your phone number and your name and people call you. My message says, "Hi, my name is Mark, and I'm real hot tonight, so call me and I'll burn you." Get it? Call me and I'll burn you. Have you ever

been burned by somebody? "Call me and I'll burn you." Think about it. I just fuck with people. I don't do it to meet any of them. I just do it to fuck with people. I've met a few of the people. They're all freaks. They're old or they're ugly.

By age twenty, Mark had been damaged by ongoing and consistent rejections and failures. He claimed that his HIV infection was intentional: "I wanted it to happen; it is just another example of my fucking up." Mark lived an ephemeral adolescence both hostile and grotesque. He experienced a development characterized by rebellion and premature separation, by derangement of the senses, with older adults who enacted a caricature of "love." He lived with alternating attacks of anger and depression; his everyday existence a constant challenge to body and spirit. No pattern of harmony was established. His life had been a consistent plunge deeper into the destructive "pit" of street life. HIV infection was just another less immediate threat. As a result and in response, Mark became an alchemist in an effort to change the reality of his situation through self-medication, and through continued impersonal sexual and criminal activity. After he put his cat out, again, he only had himself to look after.

Chapter 11

"A Different Future": Ana

The eyes may be steady with that Athenian look
that answers terror with stillness, or they may be quick
with a purely infatuate being. Almost always
the eyes hold on to an image
of someone recently departed or gone a long time ago
or only expected . . .

The eyes are not lucky.
They seem to be hopelessly inclined to linger.

They make additions that come to no final sum.
It is really hard to say if their dark is worse than their light,
their discoveries better or worse than not knowing,

but they are the last to go out,
and their going out is always when they are lifted.

–Tennessee Williams, *The Eyes,* 1956

Ana was a twenty-one-year-old, "strictly dickly" (heterosexual) woman born to Caribbean parents. She lived in a similar social world as known to Ethan, Jared, Lisa, and Mark, but on the East Coast. Her parents never married, and they separated soon after she was born. Her father lived in the Caribbean where he had four sons with a second common-law wife. Ana had a sister from her mother's relationship with another man in the United States. Ana was bilingual and spoke with a Boriqua accent, alternating between Spanish and English. She spoke with passion and intention, and was street-smart. She was tall, of medium build, with an athletic frame. She wore bright, tight-fitting bodysuits cut low in the front and accentuating her cleavage. She also wore a gold necklace with a prominent brown evil eye pendant, in remembrance of her deceased brown-eyed baby boy. She used bright red lipstick. When she smiled, crooked teeth were evident. She sucked her thumb up until a few months before her twenty-first birthday, "no shame in my game." She was getting braces to straighten her teeth. She was preoccupied with her appearance, having a manicure, pedicure, and facial on a weekly basis. She carried herself with confidence, but her face was worn, and she looked older than her actual age. Ana was raised by her mother in a rough urban neighborhood. Drug dealing and gang violence were commonplace. After continual difficulties with her mother, she left home and lived for years with girlfriends or male lovers and their families. She eventually found an apartment of her own where she lived with an infant daughter born in 1994. Ana did not attend high school, but wanted to take the GED equivalency test. Besides losing her son to AIDS in infancy, she had two abortions while a teenager. Ana recalled her own mother's unsuccessful abortion attempt and her subsequent birth.

> She left home when she got pregnant with me. I hear all sorts of stories about how she took a bunch of stuff to abort me. She didn't want to have a baby. My grandmother used to lock her out of the house because the man my mother was with would call her a whore and tell my grandmother not to let her into the house. This is while she was carrying me. Once I was born, that started the whole fight over who would take me. . . . She made a mistake in opening up her legs. She said he forced her, but I don't think so. She made a mistake. I don't blame either one of them. They were young. I've gotten over that. Besides, I'm here now!

Ana had troubles at school from an early age. She was accused of dressing provocatively during both elementary and junior high school, and she was assigned a male counselor. She identified this counselor as the only male role model she had in her life. She would go on trips and vacations with the counselor and his family. He was her "friend and therapist" for two years. During their therapy sessions, Ana recalled memories from earlier childhood that haunted Ana into her young adulthood.

There was a death when I was younger, in the apartment where we lived. A baby died and I felt that it was my fault. The landlord was taking in money for drugs, and my mother had a girlfriend that needed a place to stay. She had a little girl and a little boy. The little boy was only a couple of months old. My mother told her, "You have to put the baby in bed with you because it's cold in the apartment, it's below zero outside, and there's no heat because the landlord uses the money for drugs. You have to give the baby body heat." So the stupid bitch went dancing and left the baby in a little plastic tub on top of the table in the kitchen with the oven on. . . . The next day the baby was dead. I felt guilty that the baby died because I heard the baby cry, but I went back to sleep. I was eight years old around this time, and my bedroom was near the kitchen. A while later, I heard him cry again. Everybody was sleeping; I didn't want to wake my mother up, so I went to make him a bottle. I was old enough to do it, so I made the bottle. I put it on top of the table and I went to pick up the baby and the baby was a block of ice. He was dead. I really didn't hear him crying the second time—that was just my imagination. The first time I felt like maybe he was really crying and I could have saved him, so I always felt guilty. My counselor told me that it wasn't my fault, that I was a little girl, and that it was in God's hands.

Divine providence and "fate" became Ana's explanation for—and only comfort during—her subsequent troubles. She held God partly responsible for her helplessness, but God was also "there" for her and her children in moments of extreme crisis. Ana was physically developed by age twelve. She recalled that she was sexually active early. Her mother refused to get her birth control devices, hoping to discourage her behaviors.

I was fourteen. It was hard for my mother to realize that her child was not a baby anymore. I was having sex since I was thirteen and she didn't know it. The reason I say sex is because it wasn't love; it wasn't. Now that I'm older, I know it wasn't. I was looking for love in all the wrong places. I needed my mother's love and my father's love, and my father had never been there for me. I didn't have a male figure, so I was always looking for a father, I guess. These guys did not know my problems, but they knew I was vulnerable. They would take advantage of that. They fed on that. That's what got me into trouble, sleeping around and not knowing that I had to protect myself, and not taking care of myself. I got gonorrhea once. They talked about AIDS when I got gonorrhea—you could get AIDS and all. "Do you know about protection?" It went in one ear and out the other.

Ana blamed her mother for not helping her protect herself. She also recognized her mother's limitations.

I feel some of this is her fault in a way because she didn't educate me. She was so ignorant herself. When she found out that I wasn't a virgin, they asked her at Planned Parenthood to get me birth control protection. They wanted to sit us down and give us counseling and tell us about diseases and stuff. She said, "No, what do you want to give her birth control for? So she can be going around fucking everybody?" She slapped me and took me out of there by my hair. We went home and that was the end of the story. I hate her for that.

After this experience, Ana knew she could never again ask her mother for advice or help. However, she protected herself in other ways. Ana carried a knife and sometimes a gun for protection when she went out into the neighborhood. Throughout her adolescence she was involved in street fights with other girls, and she often had boyfriends who were drug dealers or involved in other illegal activities. She began running away from home at age thirteen.

I ran away from home at thirteen. I ran away from home a couple of times. I remember I didn't run away too far, a couple of blocks from where I lived. It was because I was dating this older guy, and he had me hypnotized. He had me wrapped around his little finger. He was my first crush. I was still a virgin and he was always trying to get me into bed, always, always, always. He never gave up. One day, he tried to rape me and I stabbed him. I got away. He didn't succeed. He has a scar on his back, and even after that I still kept talking to him. I would see this guy and my knees would start to shake, that's how scared I was of him, because he physically abused me. And my mother went looking for me; she knew I was there. She found me and took me back home, and promised things would change and she would sit down and talk to me instead of beating me and stuff. Because every time I would do something bad, instead of her sitting me down and explaining why she didn't want me to do something, she would just grab the broomstick, the mop, a wire—whatever she could find—and hit me. She would call me a bitch and a whore. She was mentally abusive. I guess that's what her mother put her through. She was just replaying what they did to her on me. I don't think she consciously meant it because after she would do it, she would start crying and felt bad and stuff. That would confuse me even more.

Ana did not have sexual intercourse with this man. Instead, she lost her virginity to Miguel about the same time. Unable to tolerate an unstable home, and due to the difficulties with her mother, Ana grew up on the street moving from one to another of her girlfriends' homes.

I used to stay at a lot of girlfriends' houses. I lived from house to house—any girlfriend who would take me home with her, I would go. Until her mother would get fed up and say, "She's a runaway; she's got to get out of the house."

Over the next six years, she moved from place to place and juggled many short-term relationships with men. All of these relationships had similar characteristics. Most involved physical abuse. When her boyfriend discovered she was not a virgin, he beat her.

When he found out I wasn't a virgin anymore, he beat me. He stood with me waiting for me to give myself to him and I never did. I went and gave myself to Miguel. I think that's why I did it because I knew it would get him mad. I did it for the first time when I was thirteen; I got pregnant and had an abortion. My mother never found out about the first abortion. I never saw Miguel again after the time we did it. It was just something that happened. . . . Then we bumped into each other again, started dating, and I stood with him. We got engaged and everything. But it didn't work out because all he wanted to do was sell drugs. I wanted to get off the coin and get a job. He didn't listen. I was living with him in his mother's house. They were driving me crazy.

She lived with Miguel and his mother for over a year, again became pregnant, and had a second abortion. Miguel was sent to jail for drug sales. While Ana was still living with Miguel's mother, she took another lover. Miguel's mother caught Ana with her new lover and threw her out of her home. Ana knew she could not go to her own mother's home, so she went to a youth shelter. She described the experiences that followed.

> I was there for a couple of days. I was so young. They always try to get the younger ones out of there quick because there are a lot of druggies in there and hookers. It is a crazy place. They didn't have rooms available at that time. I was sleeping on a floor mat, but there was a roof over my head. I was warm and I was safe, and it was better than being out on the street. I had run away before, and I knew how it was to be out on the streets. I didn't want to be out there. After the shelter, they sent me to a group home for girls thirteen to sixteen. They called my mother, and asked for a house investigation. They wanted to investigate my mother's house. They saw my mother's house. It was beautiful; you could eat off her floor. Just because the house is nice that doesn't mean you're not being abused. They sent me back home, the motherfuckers. I ran away again two months later, because I went back to the same shit. I ran away and this time it was for good. I never went back.

Ana stayed with a girlfriend for a short period of time, had a new boyfriend named Will, and moved into his apartment. As was her pattern, she would make a new boyfriend, move in with him and usually his mother, eventually get involved with someone else, and move on. She emphasized that she always paid rent when she stayed with her boyfriends. Drugs played a major role in the lives of her partners, and while Ana was a regular marijuana user, she avoided the harder drugs that were easily available.

> I met this other guy [Will] and I was living with him in his apartment that he had as a stash house, where they would keep the drugs, the money and bottles of crack and stuff—the coke and dope and everything. You name it, he was dealing it. I was never one to be turned on to drugs, thank goodness. God, because I always had so much around me. If I had been weak on that point, I would have probably ended up a junkie. It was there for the taking, and they were willing and would have given it to me. I always said, "No, no, no." Pot was the only thing I ever did—marijuana. Because my mother smoked marijuana so it was around me at the house. My first joint was with my mother. She thought I was already getting high, so she said, "If you're going to do it, you're going to do it with me."

By age sixteen, Ana had already had a number of sexual partners. She rarely had protected intercourse during her adolescence.

> Once in a while, I had a guy offer to put on a condom. Most guys wouldn't offer. If they didn't offer, I didn't think anything of it. I really didn't care. I guess I didn't value myself as much as I should have. If I was more educated and valued myself, I wouldn't have gone to bed with all those guys that I went to bed with. I wouldn't have opened my legs as easily as I used to. If they took me to the movies or bought me dinner, I thought I owed them something. I felt like I had to go to bed with them. I felt real bad growing up. . . . It starts at home. It's the mother and father's responsibility to make you feel loved, To educate you and make you feel like you don't have to go out there looking for anything, to let you know that you're looking for love in the wrong places.

Ana, like David and Lisa, differentiated her behaviors, and the rationale for her actions, from others her age. She also described her longing for love and fear of being alone.

> I had a lot of friends that went to bed with older men for money and always invited me. I never had a reason to do that,

so I would say, "No, I'm not interested." I guess I did things that weren't as bad as what they were doing, but were bad. I was going to bed with anybody to feel loved—not for exchange of money but just to feel wanted and loved because I didn't care who it was for that one night. I didn't care. I would wake up the next morning and feel dirty. It was better than being alone that night.

Ana worked several retail store jobs to earn money. During the time she lived with Will, she also baby-sat for Sandy. Sandy was a female friend who always seemed to have a lot of money. Sandy told Ana that she also could make big money in her line of work, but was not specific about her profession. Sandy invited Ana to come see for herself.

I put on a pair of jeans and some sneakers. I looked awful and I'm walking down the street and I'm getting all these whistles and comments. No matter what I put on, it's the same; I could be a nun. So I went there and as soon as I walked in, everybody was all eyes on me. There were a lot of older ladies. I was the youngest one in the place. I see the girls dancing topless, I'm like, "Oh my God, she's a stripper." I said, "Sandy, why didn't you tell me?" I said, "I wouldn't mock you for doing it, but I could never get up there and do something like that. My God are you crazy?" She said, "It's not that bad, the money is good, nobody touches you unless you let them, and it's all up to you how far it goes. You're in control." I said, "Yes, all right, whatever." The bouncer comes over to talk with me. He wants me to dance there because he knows he's going to drag in a lot of customers and make money with me. He asks me, "What's your name?" I said, "Fate," because that's my street name; everybody calls me that. He says, "Well, Fate, Sandy tells me your interested in dancing. Are you considering it?" I said "Yes, I'm considering it because I really need the money, but I don't think I have the nerve to get up there and do it." He said, "Well it's going to be hard, but you'll get over it because it goes away." I said, "Right. All these men, showing them my body—I can't." He said, "You're beautiful; you'll make a lot of money. These older ladies, you see them doing the things they're doing, they're doing it because they are old and ugly. They have to do that. You're beautiful; men will take their wallets out of their pockets and hand it to you. Just give them a little; you don't have to take it very far. Take it as far as you want to take it. You are in control." The same as Sandy said.

Ana became a stripper for the money. She described her first night in the job.

So I got up on stage and I started crying, in front of everybody. I was trying to dance and my body felt so stiff and my hands were so sweaty and my heart was pounding. I started crying. The bar was packed and I felt so embarrassed. The bouncer asked me "Are you all right? Do you want to get off?" One of the guys there was a lawyer. He was so cute, so nice to me. He was sitting right next to the stage. He says, "What's the matter, sweetheart? We don't bite in here." He made me loosen up a little and he started throwing all this money at me. I started thinking about all the stuff I could do with the money, and the fear went away.

Ana danced at a number of clubs on the East Coast over the next four years. To earn extra money, she also stripped at bachelor parties, which paid more. Ana defended stripping as a legitimate way to make money, and explained differences between clubs.

It's a shame that topless dancers have such a bad reputation. They are really straight most of the places. The places where they have their ho's and stuff as junk bags are run-down places.

About the time she began stripping, Ana remembered instances of sexual abuse that she had apparently repressed. She went for counseling, and read books and watched movies about sexual abuse and suppressed memories.

I would have nightmares about a little girl crying, "Don't touch me." I didn't know the little girl was me. When I was

> 16–I had already started dancing–I bumped into a man. He was a friend of the family that my mother would leave me with. His wife was supposed to take care of me, but she would go to work and leave me with her husband and kids. I remember telling his daughter, "Your daddy touched me in my private spot," and her telling me, "My daddy would never do something like that to you. It was probably by mistake, he was just playing with you. My daddy loves you, like you were his own daughter." She said, "He played with me like that; it was okay." I figured she's older than me; she knows better so it's okay. I was too scared to go to my mother and talk to her because I didn't have that kind of relationship with my mother. So I kept it to myself. I thought I had it with nightmares and dreams, and thought it was done. . . . Then I ran into him. I'm looking at the dirty old man. I'm like, "God, I know it's him."

She confronted him and confirmed and corroborated her suspicions that the man had molested her when she was a child. She also learned that the man's son had also had intercourse with her when she was seven. She associated her sexual problems with her earlier experiences of abuse.

> I didn't know why I was so shy about my body and why when boyfriends would ask me to get into a certain position, I would feel like it was dirty and like I was being abused. When they would play with me and pin me down to the bed and I was being held down, I would feel like I was suffocating and I wanted them to get off. I would do anything to save myself. I would stab at anybody or anything just to get them off me. I always wondered why I got these attacks. It was because of that.

While Ana danced at clubs and saved money, Will continued to deal drugs. Eventually, Will was arrested, prosecuted, and sent to prison. Ana started looking for another lover, but this time she wanted to find someone with money: "I wanted a boyfriend with a fine car, to take me out–wine me, dine me, and 69 me." One day, Ana and a friend went to buy marijuana at four o'clock in the morning, and while walking in the rain, they met Devon who was driving a luxury car with friends. Ana gave him her phone number, and she saw him the next day.

> We went to his friend's house. We're hanging out there, he likes to do blow [cocaine] once in a while, so they were all doing what they do, and I was doing what I do. Instead of going home that night because we were all messed up, we slept there. We slept together; we just held each other that night. If he would have tried something, he wasn't going to get anything because I wanted to feel clean. We hung with each other, and ever since that night, we've been together. He's my baby's father. I had a son from him, my little boy, and I have my daughter now. That's when I found out I was HIV positive, with my son from him. My little boy got PCP pneumonia, and that's how he died. He was six months old when he died.

She considered herself in a common-law marriage with Devon, referring to him as her husband and his mother as her mother-in-law. He was different from other men she dated, "He had class and he knew how to treat a woman. I wasn't really in love with him, but I loved everything about him." She grew to love him more than any of her other partners. Nevertheless, during a period when they were estranged, she had an affair with a man from work who she believed infected her. Over the years, she would "cheat" on Devon and he would "cheat" on her. Ana continued to strip while she lived with Devon, up until she got pregnant with their son at age seventeen. She considered having another abortion.

> I already had two abortions, and I regretted them both. I didn't want to have another abortion because the two abortions I had really messed up my head. Actually, the first one, the baby was four months already, and in my stomach I felt the baby move. After I had the abortion, I found out how they kill them. If I had known all the information, I would not have gone through with the abortion. I think if I would have kept the baby at thirteen, it would have been tough, but things would have been a lot different. A lot of the things I went through I wouldn't have gone through. I learned to leave things the way they are, and accept them the way they come. If they come that

way, God has something in mind. You could change your whole life, the way you're going, by one little thing you do different. I think if I would have kept that baby–that was Miguel's baby–I would have stood with Miguel. I wouldn't have jumped from man to man.

Ana did not have another abortion. Instead, she quit stripping, and Devon supported them with the money he made as a driver for a high-level drug dealer. Ana recalled in detail when she learned her HIV status.

> I didn't know anything. I had been tested and it was negative when I was pregnant for my son at seven months. I figured, "Well I'm negative, great." Then the doctors called me, my husband, and my mother-in-law into a big room. We're all thinking, "Oh no." I could see my mother-in-law's face, like "Oh God, no." She works with HIV children at the hospital and she knows the process. She knows how they tell you so she already knew. I guess she did not want to worry us so she says, "Devon, calm down," telling my husband to calm down. I'm looking at him and he's real scared. He says, "Oh God, Mom, don't tell me," telling his mother, "Don't tell me what they're going to tell us." They took us into a room and we all sat down. They're saying, "We found out what it is" and they're taking their sweet time telling us. I guess it's not easy for them to give people that kind of news. My husband is very impatient, so he says, "Whatever it is, tell us." They said "Your son has full-blown AIDS," and Devon started scream-ing. He said "Oh no, Ma I don't want to die, Ma!" He got down on his knees and started crying. I felt bad because I'm sitting there watching him, and he didn't come to me. He thought of himself. I couldn't think about him. I really didn't care about him and I didn't care about me. I didn't care if I was going to die or whatever. I couldn't stop thinking about my little baby that was lying there helpless and there was nothing I could do. I started crying. I sat there crying, and Devon was on the floor screaming, "I don't want to die; I don't want to die" to his mother. I got up and left because I couldn't take it. I could hear in the background people telling him and his

mother, "You have to understand that now all she [Ana] can think about is her son." I went to the baby, talking to him and telling him not to leave me. How sorry I was. That I didn't know, and if I would have known, I wouldn't have brought him into this world to suffer. It hurt more and more as I looked at him. He was connected to all these machines, and I knew he was going to die. He had full-blown AIDS, and at that moment, I wanted to die. I wanted the whole world to cave in and for the ground to open up and swallow me. But, it would not happen, it wasn't that easy.

She stayed away from everyone whom she loved. She did not go home to Devon, but stayed at a girlfriend's house for an extended period. She felt guilty about abandoning her baby in the hospital. She increased her drinking and marijuana use, both were available for "free" from friends. She developed "bags under her eyes," and "lost a lot of weight."

I really lost it. I started hanging out and the baby wasn't even dead yet. I couldn't go to the hospital anymore. I was in denial, and I couldn't deal with it. My husband was upset because I wasn't there for my baby while he was in the hospital. I feel guilty now too. They say that when people are going, they have a choice, their spirit can see themselves laying there, and they see you suffering, and you want them back. If you want them back strong enough, they'll come back. I don't know if that is the way it really is, but I believe that it is. I feel bad because maybe I didn't want him bad enough so he didn't stay. I also look at it this way, "If it's not time for you to go, God won't take you." I feel that maybe God just knew that it was time for him to go.

Initially, Devon's concern was only for himself until he tested negative. Then, his attention turned to his son. Throughout, little concern was shown for Ana.

I was scared. I thought that my life was over. "I'm going to die." I'd heard of people lasting years, but I wasn't thinking about anybody else. I was thinking about myself. I knew that I was sick, and I thought I was going to die. My son is laying in the hospital, and he's going to die. My husband was negative. I felt guilty thinking that he didn't love me, and that he didn't want to be with me anymore. Even though he was telling me different, I thought he was lying. I thought he was pitying me, and I don't want pity. I didn't want pity. I was scared, and I wanted to feel my baby, and I couldn't hold him and feel him. I was staying at my girlfriend's house, and she has a newborn son. I would hold him, and smell him, and feel like it was my baby, but it wasn't the same. He didn't smell like my baby and he didn't feel like my baby. He wasn't my baby.

While living at her girlfriend's place, Ana's life "hit bottom."

My girlfriend would sleep in the living room, and I would just lock myself in her room and stay in there. I liked being around her because she would not bring up the sickness. She knew—I told her—and she wouldn't bring up the baby. At this time she didn't know exactly what he was sick from, but she knew that he was dying and what I was going through. She didn't know what it was. I was totally bugging out. I was bugging out. I would go downstairs to get a bag of weed, go back upstairs, smoke in her room, and lock myself in there and watch the soap operas. I would come out of the room at about eight o' clock at night, take a shower, get dressed, and go out and party. I wasn't dancing because I couldn't take the pressure. The guys and the men, they made me sick.

She distinguished between the men who paid to see her strip and Vincent, the man she saw while separated from Devon.

I wasn't going home to Devon. One day he beat me because I hadn't been home for weeks. He said, "Where the hell have you been?" I was seeing Vincent and I was sleeping with Vincent. I kept telling Vincent, "I think I am pregnant." He said, "Well, it's not from me." We used condoms, and I said, "I didn't say it was from you. If I'm pregnant, it's my husband's." . . . Meanwhile, my son's still alive. I beeped my husband, and he said, "Get your ass over here; the baby is going to die; he doesn't have much longer to live. They think he is going to die today." I thought, "Oh my God." I jumped on the train. I had had a rough night and I hadn't slept. I had on the same clothes from the day before. I got a bag of weed and rolled up a blunt [joint]. I told my girlfriend, "Bye, I'll see you. The baby is going to die. I want to be there when he passes away."

Ana described the scene at the hospital. Devon was on his way to the hospital when the baby died. Ana was especially grateful that she was with the baby when he passed away.

The baby was hooked up to so many machines. I could not hold him, so I talked to him. I believe the person's spirit can hear you before it leaves the body. So, I talked as fast as I could before my baby's spirit left him. I could see it starting to leave on the machine because the machine started to beep slower and slower. I told him how sorry I was that he had to suffer. I loved him, even though I couldn't always be there. I told him all the things I'd kept in my heart. Then the machines stopped, and I knew he was gone.

The pain she experienced upon her son's death lessened when she had another child.

Maybe that all happened for a reason. Now I have a beautiful little girl. I don't know if she is going to be positive yet, but so far two of her tests came out negative. If she turns out to be negative, I feel like my son died for a reason. He died so I could have a healthy baby. God knows that if he had stayed alive and was sick, I wouldn't have tried for another baby. Maybe God said, "She deserves a healthy baby; I'll take this one from her because he's only coming into this world to suffer. I'll give her another one." I feel lucky because while the baby was sick in the hospital, I was already three weeks pregnant with my daughter.

For young women who lose children to AIDS, the reorganization of their lives was a lengthy and difficult process (Welle, Luna, and

Rotheram-Borus, 1996c). The guilt associated with "causing" their infants' death was often insurmountable. Ana's experiences, and to a degree, Lisa's experiences illustrate how the process of living with HIV differs for women with children compared to those who are childless like Marie. Ana believed she could not force the transition, as she explained when she examined a photograph of herself looking especially gaunt.

> That picture was taken when my son was dying. God I was wasted when that picture was taken! I had a good time that night. Everybody knew I was really suffering. Guys would buy me drinks in the bar. Everyone knew what was going on, they would ask "How's your baby?" I would say, "He's dying." I would fake a big happiness smile and we'd go out and dance our asses off. It was all pretend. I really wanted to die.

Her daughter's birth just months after her son's death eased her pain and was a life elixir.

> She's a Pisces. People pick her up to hold her when they're down. It's like she's medicine for people.

Ana received special health and social services for youths living with HIV. She brought her daughter to HIV support groups where group members took turns holding and looking after her. She was proud of her daughter, and developed a will to live for her benefit. Ana was happy that she had another child to love and care for.

> I'm glad I had her, even though everybody was against it. I used to smoke a lot of weed because I'd get so depressed and down. It was the only thing that would take the edge off, that would give me any peace. But now that I have her, I don't smoke as much. I'm not as depressed as before. Really, she's the only thing in life that can take the pain away.

Ana attended HIV groups once or twice a week, and decided she wanted to finish her GED and go to college. She started to "take life more seriously." Spiritual practices played an increasing role in Ana's coping with past troubles. While her religious mother engaged in spiritual practices at home, Ana understood but did not share in these same practices. She did not attend church, but prayed often. She cited periods in her life when God was her only source of conciliation.

When her son was born, Ana placed a gold cross and chain around his neck for protection. His godmother gave the baby an "evil eye," that the baby wore from birth. When the baby died, Ana took the eye and cross off her son and kept them. When her daughter was born, Ana put her son's jewelry on her new baby.

> I couldn't decide whether to have her wear it. One day, I went ahead and put them on her. Something weird happened. I put the chain on her, and the eye and the cross, and she wore it all day. Then, when I was getting her bottle ready, all of the sudden she handed me the chain in her hand. It was kind of hanging off her hand. I thought, now how did that fall off her? How come it fell into her hand? Is she trying to give it back to me, like, "This isn't mine, Mommy?" I decided that was kind of creepy. After that, I put the eye and the cross together, and I wear them. I have never taken them off. Besides, she has her bracelet for now, which has African colors. I think it's the colors of one of the saints, and the fist for protection.

After reflecting upon her daughter's responses to the son's protective items, Ana realized they were not appropriate for her daughter. She decided that she should wear the son's protective items, and assigned meaning to her daughter's rejection of the jewelry.

> I should wear it. It's for me. She really had nothing to do with him, although I will tell her all about her brother. I'm the one that has the memories of him, anyway, not her. I don't need to put all of that on her. Hopefully, she will have *a different future*.

Ana reaffirmed a connection to her dead son and prayed that the same tragedy would not repeat with her daughter. She believed that the responsibility for her son's death was ultimately "on her," and was not something to pass on to her daughter.

Ana's beliefs about death were influenced by her religious background and were supported by her folk spiritual practices. She was convinced that premature death was a reward for a life of extreme suffering.

> The way I see it, people who have suffered a lot leave this life early. This world is hell; we're all living in hell right now. Those people who have already gone through enough hell, they die young. They get to go on up to heaven before the rest of the people. People who live to their sixties or seventies, you know they've had it easier. God is making them stick out more years to really experience things.

Ana wished aloud that she would have more time to live, to help with her daughter's education, and to complete her own personal projects.

> I just hope I live another three years at least. I'm getting braces on this year, and they're telling me it's going to take three years to correct this overbite. Can't you just see me finally getting my teeth fixed, and then just die? Or die before they ever get straightened out? I couldn't take it! Going to my grave wearing braces!

Ana recounted one experience that provided her with a spiritual framework to understand how and why others mistreated her. It also provided meaning to her circumstances.

> This one witchcraft man in our neighborhood, he came up to me one day on the street, and he said, "Ana, I bet people get jealous of you. I bet they just leave you alone, and think you think you're so big." I was shocked, because it's true; most people just leave me alone. They don't like my attitude or something. He said that was because of who I was in a past life. He said that we go around over and over again, making the same mistakes over and over until we get it right. I believe that. He said in my past life, I was like a mistress, not exactly a prostitute, but like a Madame, and I didn't let anybody mess with me. He says people in this life, they pick that up from me–that I had those kind of involvements–and they stay away because things from way far back in the past are still hanging around me.

Although Ana had undergone individual and group counseling at the HIV Youth Program that focused on her troubles in adolescence, her encounter with this neighbor provided special understanding. She was able to distance herself from her past experiences and identity while acknowledging their current impact on her life. Her neighbor's opinions that her strengths and insecurities were a reflection of reincarnation and "karma" made sense to her. Seeing purpose in mistakes, Ana considered HIV to be something that she was supposed to learn from in order to prevent further suffering in her next life. She learned practical lessons from her life experiences, and she believed they were educational rather than punitive in nature. Not long after encountering the "witchcraft" man on the street, Ana utilized the reincarnation philosophy to interpret a dream she considered initially disturbing, but later life-affirming.

> We were in a car. My baby son was with me. He was talking to me, asking me to bring him home. I couldn't understand it because when he died, he was too young to talk. So I feel he was talking to me from the afterlife, to let me know that he's okay, and that I can bring this new baby home instead of him. It was his way of talking to me from the other side, telling me to relax in this life, and keep living.

Ana curtailed her smoking, prayed to keep her hopes up, and looked for positive news in the media about HIV and AIDS. Like Ethan, she was getting close to "aging out" of the HIV Youth Program and was hesitant about repeating her whole history to new providers. She summarized her life thus far and her plans for the future. She had developed a coherent version of her life story and fate.

> I've had a pretty good life. What gets me mad is just when I finally got it together, just after I found this man that I'm going to stay with, that I was happy with, I changed my ways. Before I met Devon I had stopped jumping around, jumping into bed with everybody because I started to care about myself more, and I learned how to deal with problems, understanding why my mother treated me like that, why this man abused me and his son had sex with me, why I was running away, and how

men are. I grew up. . . . I feel like I'm in a race against time. I'm trying to do everything before I die. There are places I haven't been to. I want to travel and I want to do this and do that. You feel like you have to rush and do everything because you don't know when you are going to go. It's kind of stupid when you think about it; you feel that way because you're HIV positive. You're going to die anyway. Everybody does, so it's funny that you panic because you have a disease and you're going to die. You're going to die regardless. . . . I want to be alone now. I want to concentrate on my daughter and school and positive things in my life. I don't need the stress. I don't need to clean up after anybody else, just me and my daughter. Those are the stages you go through when you find out. You're in denial, and then it's limbo—your life just goes on hold. You just get out of control and you do destructive things. After a while it starts to sink in and you start taking life more seriously. You start thinking, "How much time do I have left to do this?" . . . But, I don't regret none of this. If I could take anything back, the only thing I would take back is the HIV infection. That would be the only thing I would take back. Everything else I've learned from. It was a learning experience, and it helped me grow. It made me a better woman and I'll be a better mother for my daughter. I don't know how much time I'll have to be a mother to her, but I'll make the best of it.

Chapter 12

"Everything Will Fall into Place": Rose

I met an apparition and so did she.
She was lovely as ever and even more fragile than ever
and her eyes
were blind-looking.
I found myself unable to think and speak a little.
"What have you been doing lately, Helen?"
Indifferently she said: "When you take pills around the clock
what you do is try to get money to pay the drugstore."

                                    —Tennessee Williams, *Night Visit,* 1977

Rose was a twenty-two-year-old, heterosexual female who described herself as "no race in particular," but "passed" for many. She
grew up in a multiracial household, speaking fluent Spanish, English, and Portuguese. She was the second of three children. She was
raised a Catholic, but practiced her "own kind of religion." Rose
thought most religions were prejudiced and hypocritical, but occasionally she attended family functions held at liberal churches. She
had a Southern accent to her voice, and spoke with a heavy lisp as a
result of a childhood automobile accident. She had reconstructive
facial surgeries from ages eight to twelve following the accident.

Rose was light-skinned, and accentuated her looks with elaborate
hairstyles. She wore makeup to cover superficial facial scars; her
facial features were slightly asymmetrical as a result of her accident.
She was short in stature, walked carefully, and was frail looking.
Like Ana, she appeared to be years older than her actual age. She
frequently wore stretch-leggings covered by oversized sweaters.
After her father deserted the family a number of years ago, she had
daily contact with a close, large network of relatives, including
cousins, aunts and uncles, and grandparents.

Rose believed that she was infected by blood transfusions following the accident in the early 1980s when she was still a child. The accident was serious, and she suffered multiple injuries. She lost a lot of blood. She described her time in hospital.

> I was in the hospital for two months. I was in intensive care for two weeks because I almost died. When I came home, I was in a half-body cast. When I was in the hospital the children I shared a room with. . . . would look because I had stitches all across my face and my hair was all bloodied and tangled and matted. One girl, she had all these games. She kept the curtains around her bed closed because I guess looking at me repulsed her or something. She made me feel bad. In the beginning, I couldn't even open my eyes, they were closed. A lot of the time, they kept me in the room by myself.

At the time, concerns about HIV infection were uncommon.

> When I lived there, at that time, they were not checking the blood, and hepatitis and AIDS were in the blood. They say you get yeast infections when you're exposed to HIV. You tend to get more yeast infections. I used to get a lot of yeast infections when I was a child after I got out of the hospital. They asked me if I was having sex! A child. Not!

Rose supported herself with money from a substantial legal settlement she received following the accident. She found out that she was HIV infected years later while in high school.

> When I went to high school, a nurse said I should go to this clinic so I went. First I tested for hepatitis, because my boyfriend had it so they tested me. But I had a different type than he did. He had A, and I had B. So I started seeing the doctor for that. Then he asked me if I wanted to take the HIV test. I thought, "Yeah, okay." I really didn't think anything of it [laughs]. They told me I was positive and I said, "What?" I was shocked and depressed, and they put me in the hospital for a couple of weeks. They thought I might kill myself or something [laughs]. I thought about it, but I could never go through

with it because I don't like taking pills and so I couldn't over-
dose. I didn't have any pills anyway! Then they thought I
might cut my wrists, but I can't see myself doing any of those
things. While I was in the hospital, I was real depressed so I
called up my boyfriend and he was all worried [laughs]. He
thought he had to get himself checked out. I told my mother
and then I told my best friend. They were all supportive of me.
I was lucky.

Rose was selective of who she informed of her HIV status.

Just my family and my best friend knows; two of my friends
know. I don't tell people too much because sometimes people
are so ignorant. They don't know what to say or how to act,
and they are real prejudiced. The people I have told–I have
been basically lucky–they've been supportive and understanding.

She changed her dating and substance use practices after learning of
her HIV infection.

I used to have a lot of boyfriends and I used to hang out all
the time. I wasn't one for drinking or using drugs, even though
at one time in my life I did. But I stopped that. I used to smoke
reefer and I used to do coke. I wasn't gaining nothing from it,
and it wasn't doing anything for me. It was dragging me down.
That's before I found out. I stopped one day. I just stopped.
People don't find it that easy. I see a lot of my friends, and they
still smoke reefer and do coke. After I found out, for health
reasons, I stopped. Because hepatitis is a liver disease and
drugs make it worse.

She recalled her initial reaction to the diagnosis.

At first, being HIV positive, it's a death sentence. When I
found out I had to make big adjustments. It's hard to face it and
not look at the downside of things–you're going to die one day.
First, you have to be supportive of yourself before you look for
support. It helps to get support, but first you have to be positive
and think positive. You have to be ready to deal with anything.

Rose identified the biggest obstacle she had to overcome living with HIV.

> Admitting it. When I found out, I was seeing a psychiatrist, a therapist, so that helped with the feelings I had. I could go to her and she helped me. That helps; definitely that helps a lot. Having a therapist before you tell anybody else about it and talking it over with them helps. Just admitting the fact that I was HIV positive, not making major changes in my life, but changing my lifestyle a bit helped so that I wouldn't injure myself anymore.

The lifestyle changes she made seemed simple, but in fact, had repercussions in other areas of her life. Ultimately, she "had to be there" for herself.

> Like not pushing myself. You have to think about other people when you have sex, and use a condom. Thinking about other people—that was the change. You have to care for yourself with a good diet. Eat better, try to get some rest, if you can, exercise. I gained a lot of weight. You have to concentrate on your health. And, I wasn't doing so well in school, and I was using HIV as an excuse. I was being lazy. I used HIV as a cop-out for many things. That's not good—using HIV as a cop-out for things. I was not doing things because I didn't really want to do them. My heart was not in it. It had nothing to do with my health. As I get older I think I see more and more. I'm still young, but I'm going through all this and I have to deal with it. I have to be strong. I have to be there for myself. If nobody else is there, at least I have myself.

Rose recalled that she began having sex at age thirteen, and had her first abortion at fourteen. She learned about sex through trial and error. Her mother, sister, and cousins never talked to her about sex although they discussed it among themselves. Rose had several sexual encounters, after which her partners gave her money—money that she did not solicit. She recognized the difference, as two of her cousins were "prostitutes." Rose's boyfriends gave her money to buy feminine clothing. Instead, she spent the money on sneakers.

She felt her rejection of passive feminine roles was healthy and helped her to stand up to boyfriends. She was glad that she was a tomboy as a child. Rose always felt closer to males than females. She had few female friends.

> I have a lot of men friends and people sometimes see me with guys and they think I'm a party girl. They don't think that you can have a relationship with a guy that's just a friendship. I am with so many guys that are my friends! Males are better friends than females. At least you don't have to worry about them talking about you, calling you names.

Rose didn't experience sexual pleasure in her early relationships, or have any sense of the pleasureable characteristics. She learned the difference between having sex and making love from Rocky her first "real" boyfriend when she was in high school. He was older, and sexually experienced. She had unprotected sex with Rocky, got pregnant, and had her second abortion at age 18. Rocky was expert at playing "mind games."

> I think that was the best choice I could have made because Rocky would have given me hell if I would have kept it. He would have made my life miserable. He tried to control me; he tried to make me feel bad, tried to make me feel like I was less than other women. He couldn't do it. . . . I'm too headstrong to let him get to me like that. . . . He couldn't infiltrate this head of mine. . . . I was really sad about how he treated me–badly. Afterward, after the abortion, he told me he would have understood it, if I would have kept the baby.

Even after she tested positive, Rocky and Rose continued to have unprotected sexual relations. Before they broke up, and a few months after Rose tested positive, Rocky said he had been tested.

> Rocky, my ex, told me he got tested and it was negative. When it came to dealing with men, they were real supportive. Before we got involved with anything I would tell them. "I think it's only fair for you to know I'm HIV positive." They would say, "I don't care. I still want to be with you." I felt lucky.

She left Rocky soon after the abortion, not because he was too controlling, but because he was involved with other women.

> He was too much. He was having many problems; he had a lot of girlfriends. This girl came to my house and she told me she was sleeping with him. I felt bad; she was telling me that she was pregnant by him and he didn't even know. He said he didn't sleep with her. The thought of him being with this girl! I looked better than her. I'm much nicer to him, and I have more intelligence. I didn't know what he saw in her. But he can stay with her because I'm not going to be there. He started it all and I didn't appreciate that. So, we can just stay friends because I'm not going to be worried about all these girls coming in my face. That wasn't the first time that happened, that a girl came to me saying she had been with him. I'm getting too old for this. I don't want to fight for guys. There are too many men in this world to fight for one. Unless you're my husband, that's different, because he's my man.

In 1993, Rose began a relationship with Rick. They knew each other a long time before they became lovers.

> I met him through one of my girlfriends. We were friends for a long time. We've been together for a year as boyfriend and girlfriend, but we knew each other for three years before that. So we're going on four years. We developed a friendship. Then when his father passed away, we started getting closer.

Even though she was dating other men, Rick waited for Rose to commit to their relationship.

> I was still seeing other guys, and Rick would get frustrated. He was the one who said, when you're ready to settle down, you let me know. He would wait for me, and that definitely takes a man; he's very patient.

Rick worked in a supermarket. She described Rick in more detail, and compared the support she received from him to that received by other young women she knew who were living with HIV.

Rick, the boyfriend I have now, I live with him and he's the father of my babies. He is very kind and loving, real support-ive. I'm lucky when it comes to a strong support system. I still keep in contact with my ex-boyfriend. My friends don't dis-criminate against me and my family is there for me. Some of the girls in the clinic, a lot of the girls are younger than me, and they have a lot of problems with their families. Their families are not as supportive.

Rick and Rose rarely used condoms during sex, and she became pregnant soon after they moved in together.

I always made him use a condom. I wasn't worried about that until we started living with each other. Even though he knew about my HIV, sometimes he would use them and some-times he would not use them. I said, "You know you have to use them—it's important to use them." But, I can't force him to do anything he doesn't want to do. Rocky, when I found out and I told him, he wore a condom once. Then he refused to wear them. I said, "You know you have to protect yourself? You know you can't do this because you're only going to hurt yourself." Unless he knew something he wasn't telling me. He said he got tested and it was negative, but I don't know if that's true or not. I used to use birth control pills. After I found out that I had hepatitis and that birth control affects your liver, the doctors strongly advised me against using birth control. So if I had sex with anybody, I tried to get them to use a condom, and that would be my birth control. With Rick, he wouldn't use anything, and I got pregnant. He said, "It's your fault, too, because you should have kept your legs crossed." I said, "You should have used a condom; now I have to deal with two brats." He said, "You shouldn't say that. God works in myste-rious ways." He said, "The way you talk, it sounds like you're not happy." I said, "I'm happy. God knows; I thank him every day, so don't even go there." I have to be very careful how I say anything.

Rick never tested for HIV.

He doesn't want to get tested. He's afraid I guess. He wouldn't be able to deal with it. I really don't push him, I mean if he does, he does, and if he doesn't—I know it takes a strong mentality to deal with that. He's already had to deal with me, and then to deal with himself. I don't know if I would be able to deal with it. God forbid if any of the kids came out with it. In time, if he wants to, he can go do it, but I'm not going to push him.

Rose was happy that she was pregnant, and distinguished between her current pregnancy and another in the past. She struggled with whether to continue the pregnancy or have an abortion, and a number of concerned others complicated her decision.

When I found out I was pregnant, I was glad because I was pregnant before and I had an abortion. So I said, "I'm pregnant now and I'm coping, so it's better for me now to keep it. If I get older, I won't be as healthy. God forbid I get sick or something and then I can't have kids." So I was three months along and I started getting really scared. I was starting to chicken out. "What if the baby gets sick?" "What if I get sick and can't take care of the baby?" All these things were going through my mind. One day I was going to keep it; the next day I wasn't. "I can't deal with this, I can't take it. I don't know if I'm ready to have a baby." I told Rick I was going to have an abortion. He was against it. I told him we really couldn't afford a baby, and the relationship was still new. But he said, "No, I want this baby." He really wanted it and we sat down and talked about it. I told him I was scared about the baby testing positive for HIV and me getting sick and not being able to take care of the baby. He told me that we would be together, and he would be there for me. We would take care of it together. I said, "Okay, I'll keep it." I guess if I was to get rid of it, I would feel bad. I talked about it with my social worker at the clinic. She wasn't saying for me to keep it or get rid of it. But she said the chances were about thirty percent that the baby would have HIV, seventy percent it would be all right. The doctor wasn't saying anything either. He wasn't trying to talk me into keeping it. He was saying, as a friend, the positive points—both negative and positive. I was real depressed for a couple of days because the decision was on me. I looked into my heart, and I didn't feel anything. I didn't know what to do! My heart was not cooperating. I couldn't feel anymore. After talking with my boyfriend I was better, like the world was lifted off my shoulders, relieved. I felt positive about my decision. Then my mother also tells me to keep it. She said she would help if I needed it–she would help. I was trying to be realistic and she had an answer for everything I said. She was really pushing me to keep it. She had advice for everything. So, I felt all right about it.

She soon learned she was pregnant with twins.

It was a shock, because I found out when I went to get my sonogram. They said to me, "Oh, you're having twins." I said, "Twins? Twins? Thank you, God. Twins, I don't believe it." I was real happy.

Knowing that her mother would help her, and in spite of health difficulties and relationship problems she had with Rick, Rose decided to carry the pregnancy to term. Rose recalled a dream she had after learning the twins could be born seropositive, develop AIDS, and die in "two years." At the time, she was deciding between having an abortion, and following her physician's advice to take AZT and have the babies, accepting her mother's offer to help raise them.

I didn't know which way to go. Everything was so extreme. Either keep two babies, or take out two babies. I felt I shouldn't, because keeping them could mean losing them later. But taking them out now, that could just be out of fear–you never know. Then my mother told me to go ahead, and she'll be there, which helped me. I still didn't know if I could handle them being sick and maybe dying. Then I had this dream. I was in this graveyard at night, I was standing in a shawl with a little baby in my arms. I was standing at this one grave, like somebody had just died. The grave was real small, so I knew it was for a baby. When I woke up, I knew I could handle it, having the babies. Because if just one of them would survive, I could handle it–even if one of them died. Let me go ahead and keep them. Maybe God will let me keep both of them, or maybe he'll just take one of them. As long as one of them makes it, I can make it, too.

Rose started prenatal AZT therapy, but struggled to maintain control of her treatment. She took exception to the AZT dosage her physician ordered. She recognized that AZT was necessary for her babies' health, but worried that it might compromise her own.

I understand they need it to be healthy when they're born. I waited to decide how to take it because I don't exactly want to get cancer myself! I want to be around to mother them, after all! They wanted me to take it three times a day, and I felt that was too much. So what I do is, I take it twice a day. Once a day ... for each of the twins, because they need it. Then I skip the third time a day because that one's for me. I don't want to take AZT for me. Besides, they're going to give me an AZT IV during the delivery.

Rose regularly read reports about HIV and AIDS developments and treatments, as well as books on childbirth and parenting. She occasionally went to the HIV clinic for group sessions, and she consistently made her appointments at a university hospital for prenatal care.

I go to see the doctor once a week and they check my blood because I'm anemic, and to see if the AZT affects it. Because AZT makes you more anemic. So they have to keep track of it. I go in for fetal evaluation once a week as well, and then prenatal once a week so the whole week is pretty busy. I hear the same thing over and over. There's nothing new that they're telling me. The only new thing is that the babies are gaining weight and growing nicely. That's good to hear. The nurse said if they keep growing at the same rate, they're going to be six pounds each; that's twelve pounds if I go full term. Oh my gosh! They're killing me now! I can't imagine when they're five or six pounds each. That's a lot.

Her pregnancy and family relationships were more significant influences in her life than were her HIV-related experiences or concerns. She had little contact with other people who were living with HIV and AIDS other than through her infrequent participation in the HIV youth groups. As her pregnancy advanced, Rose became less willing to go to support groups. She described periods of depression and the physical toll the pregnancy with twins took on her body.

> They're killing my legs. They don't let me sleep. I wake up about four or five times during the night, and I wake up every day at seven or eight o'clock. I'll be so tired I'll go back to sleep. I hate early morning appointments because I just wake up and it's so early and I'm tired. Let me go back to sleep. I'll go to the doctor another day. But I keep appointments.

Compared to other youths living with HIV and AIDS, life was relatively easy for Rose. Nevertheless, like others, she suffered physical traumas early in life, began sexual activity early, lived in subsidized low-income housing, and had power-imbalanced relationships with partners. Childbirth and motherhood were important reasons for her to live. Like many others, she could not totally ignore her HIV status. She feared repercussions, and she recognized public ignorance surrounding her infection.

> You have to learn to look at people and say to yourself, "It's okay; they're ignorant." A lot of people don't know about HIV and they have a lot to learn. They only hear the bad stuff about it—how people die from it, how many people are drug users, and how many people are homosexuals. They don't understand how other people got it, how many kids got it through their mothers, or how many people got it through their husbands or wives, or through blood transfusions.

Nevertheless, Rose was generally optimistic while still tentative about her future.

> You can't think about the future. I want to move into a better neighborhood; I want to get a car. Things like that you don't think about now. You think about them when you have the money and when you can do it. Now, you just think about today. This is what I can handle for today and this is what I'm

going to do today. I can afford this; I can't afford that. I take it one day at a time. The only thing I hope is that the babies are healthy, and that they don't have the virus. That's all I can hope for now. Everything else comes in time. *Everything will fall into place.*

Rose delivered twins boys in late 1994, Ricky Junior (after his father), and Rosario, who family members call "Rosi" (after Rick's mother). Both were born HIV negative. She started to fear that she had short-changed the babies during her pregnancy. After she returned home with the twins, she gave each double the dose of AZT that was recommended. Rose was very protective of her babies, and she rarely let them out of her sight. She insisted that everyone wash their hands before touching them.

Chapter 13

Discussion

There is yet much to be done for the lepers. Many who seem whole and sound, who are still in full enjoyment of life and liberty, are doubtless the unconscious victims of a disease that has been declared incurable by the best medical testimony of the age. The germ has been planted—it has possibly been inherited—and sooner or later it will make itself visible. The law of segregation must be enforced until the last leper has ended his miserable existence, and the survivors are delivered from the ravages of the plague. The fear of contagion and of possible infection hangs over the ill-fated Kingdom.

–Charles Warren Stoddard, *The Lepers of Molokai*, 1910

The true path was indicated upward of a century before Lord Bacon's time, by Leonardo da Vinci, in these few words: "Cominciare dall' esperienza e per mezzo di questa scoprirne la ragione." "Commence by experience, and by means of this discover the reason." In many groups of phenomena we must still content ourselves with the recognition of empirical laws; but the highest and more rarely attained aim of all natural inquiry must ever be the discovery of their causal connection.

–Alexander von Humboldt, *Cosmos: A Sketch of the Physical Description of the Universe*, 1852

Life adjustments following HIV infection were common, ranging from total isolation to full-time AIDS activism, there were many ways youths coped with their HIV status. Some middle-class young adults, for example, intentionally put themselves in public situations in which their status was disclosed to strangers that they were living with HIV or AIDS. Public exposure was a strategic part of their coping process, as these youths took risks and experienced consequences. They put themselves in positions where other people had to confront the fact they were young people living with HIV. This "in your face" stance was very much a part of their youthfulness, and is characteristic of youth culture (Luna and Rotheram-Borus, 1996b). Others became peer educators in empowerment programs or developed high profile identities as "HIV people" (Cranston, 1991; Welle, Luna, and Rotheram-Borus, 1996a; Luna and Rotheram-Borus, 1996a). Others, intentionally sought suburban environments where they lived anonymously or in isolation (Luna and Rotheram-Borus, 1997b). The social identities of youths living with HIV and AIDS in the suburbs were less determined by their infection status, and there was more variation in their time commitment to AIDS-related programs. Josh, for example, was isolated and avoided organized activities other than those necessary for his medical care. David participated in AIDS activities more often than Josh, for altruistic reasons and in order to meet a potential boyfriend who was living with HIV. HIV infection played an even more prominent role in Marie's life. She became an outspoken AIDS activist. Young women like Lisa, Ana, and Rose intentionally, or unintentionally, became pregnant, and coped with HIV as mothers. For economically disadvantaged youths or those with troubled pasts, who lacked social and economic mobility, fewer options existed. Many like Ethan and Mark, were "stuck" in "toxic" environments and lifestyles.

Some definitions are necessary to understand and appreciate how youths responded to their HIV infections. Adaptation is the ongoing process of maintaining equilibrium between individuals within and outside of their respective environments and social worlds. Adaptation as defined on the individual and psychological levels is the creation, or implementation, of a strategy to stabilize a new or rapidly changing self-concept or social identity, or to maintain equilibrium. All of the youths studied had to adapt in one way or another to their new health status, and thus they developed strategies in response. The concept of strategy is intricately linked to that of adaptation.

A strategy is a means of satisfying minimal requirements for staying alive, in two spheres. The first sphere includes all basic physiological needs, such as sustenance and protection from external threats. This sphere includes income, employment, food, and housing. For many impoverished youths living with HIV and AIDS, each day meant obtaining basic necessities for survival—often by illegal means. The second sphere is characterized by a personal or social need for a "satisfying" social life or identity, including friends, family, and sexual partners. For those living in "toxic" environments where criminal activity and substance abuse were commonplace and the population was transitory, more supportive, trusting, long-term relationships were difficult to establish or maintain. For those living in suburban areas or who had more resources at their disposal, participation in groups, functioning as peer educators, or becoming public spokespeople on HIV and AIDS gave meaning to their lives.

Coping is the psychological adjustment that occurs when adaptations must be made in behavioral routines as the result of an outside threat or a perceived change in health or social status, such as HIV infection. Coping is considered socially competent if the equilibrium experienced prior to HIV infection is maintained, or if positive life changes are made after testing HIV positive. New goals may be identified, defined, and operationalized in achievable ways. Coping is generally considered as socially incompetent if self-harmful or aggressive behaviors result, or if withdrawal or isolation occurs.

There are differences between what service providers and youths considered competent as opposed to socially incompetent ways of coping with HIV infection. For example, clinicians and service providers believed that participation in experimental HIV therapeutic regimes was indicative of proactive, positive coping. However, youths thought the same activity was representative of deferring control and responsibility to others, or "giving up." Youths and providers both believed improved dietary habits; increases in exercise; and moderations in smoking, drug, and alcohol use practices were beneficial behaviors in response to HIV infection. Providers believed that youths who withdrew, became more isolative, or avoided service programs needed to be more integrated into services, and their behavior indicated that psychological support services were necessary. Many youths employed denial of HIV status as a defense, allowing them to disavow future difficulties, and continued to concentrate on their more immediate circumstances. Those with nonprogressive HIV did not deal with their health status until anxiety following decreases in T cells occurred. "Denial as defense" was a central coping mechanism (Edelstein, Nathanson, and Stone, 1989) and was characteristic of many youths living with HIV following diagnosis.

Incompetent coping was identifiable in behaviors that were self-harmful, including continuing activities that were unprotected which could lead to reinfection. For those who had chronic substance abuse histories, it was difficult to distinguish changes in use practices as a result of HIV infection (Rotheram-Borus et al., 1994). Few chronic methamphetamine or speed users were able to curtail use without substantial assistance from social service agencies regardless of their HIV status. An economic relationship existed between drug use and sex work. Sex work enabled many to continue drug use practices, either through direct cash exchange or by bartering sex for drugs. Causal order varied; youths either engaged in sex work to support drug habits, or they used drugs to cope with their sex work. Same-sex preference and the desire for sexual partners were main reasons male youths entered sex work, thus complicating the drug-sex connection (Luna, 1994a; Luna, 1994b). Daily monetary needs of males who were dependent upon sex work for their livelihood, did not change after their HIV infection (Steward, 1991). Most continued in commercial sexual activity, and like Ethan, were susceptible to coercion when clients offered more money for unprotected sexual activities (Luna, 1994a).

At some point, all youths living with HIV desired independence and autonomy; however, paradoxically, immediately after notification, most accepted or engendered the helpless role offered by service providers. Trauma bonds were established with providers. Clinics and services became institutional parents. Personal adaptation was orchestrated and managed by the social and health care system. Most accepted the new identity and the accompanying resources that were provided, without considering the long-term consequences. For a majority of youths infected with HIV who were regular clients of the service system, the virus became the defining characteristic of their social identity. Their circumstances defined their personhood, and they were considered for all purposes *HIV-positive youths*. This identity often influenced or determined their coping and the adaptational strategies they employed, especially in urban or poverty-ridden environments. Those in suburban or rural environments, or those less connected to social or health services, had more role diversity in their lives and were able to establish more fulfilling alternative identities (Luna and Rotheram-Borus, 1997b). However, they also were more isolated and disconnected from others experiencing similar life events and the accompanying stresses. They had a more difficult time in coping as they reconciled their health status with multifaceted identities, careers, and future plans.

Five significant adaptational concerns for youths living with HIV and AIDS were identified and can be summarized.

First and most significant, adaptation to HIV status occurred concurrent with normal age-related developmental adaptations (physical, cognitive, emotional, sexual, and social). Self-expression and self-fulfilling opportunities were reduced. While most HIV infections that occurred during adolescence were considered "non-progressive" and did not immediately lead to clinical AIDS, psychological adjustments and coping, and social plans and strategies had to made based upon the realization that in the late 1980s and early 1990s life expectancy following an AIDS diagnosis was believed limited. The normal adolescent moratorium or latency period, developmental tasks, and feelings of invulnerability were either accelerated or foreclosed.

Second, outstanding past experiences or problems had to be recognized and resolved. For example, histories of severe neglect, physical and sexual abuse, violations of trust by friends or lovers, family difficulties or estrangement, substance abuse, bartering sex for drugs or commercial sex work, and issues concerning sexual preference all came into clearer focus when youths were understanding, responding, and adapting to their HIV infection. Critical life events and involvement in risk situations and settings were examined, and an understanding and explanation for HIV infection was developed. A personally relevant explanatory *"HIV Story"* became necessary not only for subsequent disclosure to family, friends, or significant others, but as a strategy for linking with relevant services and obtaining appropriate health care.

Third, the meaning of infection and how life would be affected was explored and understood, including concerns about health care, housing, financial and emotional support, and relationships. Decisions were made about disclosure. Youths decided when and to whom they would disclose their HIV status. Self-questioning occurred. Would a sexual life be possible in the future? Would a committed loving relationship be obtainable? Would isolation result?

Fourth, a determination was made about how public or private to be about HIV infection status, and impression management strategies were devised. Decisions were made regarding whether or not to adopt a public or semipublic identity as a person living with HIV or AIDS. Initially, most youths, like David, chose to live without any of their significant others knowing about their infection. The more closely tied to social or health services, the more likely youths were to adopt a more public or "out" persona as a "young person living with HIV" (Luna and Rotheram-Borus, 1997b; Welle, Luna, and Rotheram-Borus, 1996a). Service providers often inappropriately encouraged youths to come out as "HIV positive" immediately following diagnosis. Some youths were exploited for program promotion or for fund-raising purposes. The consequences of this openness was not immediately advantageous nor in the long-term best interests of the youths involved. Public and media activities, in which the identities of adolescents living with HIV were disclosed "put a face to the disease" and increased a sense of vulnerability in uninfected youths, who otherwise believed themselves invulnerable. The focus in presentations was usually on the changes that youths living with HIV had made, often using materials from their life stories, which often included substance abuse or sex work. However, these public activities created personas that some later had to carry into their complicated private lives. There were repercussions in diminished occupational opportunities, and loss of anonymity. The majority were not legally, socially, developmentally, physically, or emotionally emancipated. Even for emancipated youths who were high profile and had gone public about their HIV infection, their medical diagnosis became their social identity and would remain so for an extended time (Luna and Rotheram-Borus, 1997b).

Finally, fifth, an existential realization eventually occurred, both through explaining infection as the result of fate or destiny, or as the motivation for making spiritual growth, metaphysical development, or practical life changes. This was especially evident with Ana and Rose, who were no longer just responsible for their lives, but for their babies' lives as well. The need became more immediate to put their lives in order, to improve their existing circumstances, or to obtain spiritual comfort. The development of life-affirming future orientations depended upon the availability and accessibility of supportive services, and the resolve of youths to change the direction of their lives. Most significant, they had to feel they were worthy of better lives, and that they could accomplish the necessary changes.

Avoidance, withdrawal, and denial of HIV and AIDS were major coping reactions for youths following notification of infection. This was especially true until symptoms occurred or death became more likely. Disavowal of HIV and AIDS status must be recognized as a significant problem necessitating attention, especially as efficacious pre-AIDS treatments are developed, and in order to prevent reinfection and the infection of others.

The ways that young people were infected with HIV differed, and their available economic and social resources varied. Jared and Lisa, for example, came from different economic and social worlds. However, there were similarities in how their lives evolved and in the challenges they faced as a result of their HIV infection. For the young people studied, testing positive was an upsetting experience, and it forced them to reexamine past relationships and "taboo" activities that were difficult to incorporate into their more current identities, relationships, and peer groups. Testing HIV seropositive not only necessitated self-examination and the challenges of disclosure, but for many required efforts to reorganize their lives. Most moved to different cities shortly after testing positive, believing that life changes would be easier. At drop-in rap and support groups, they met attractive and inspiring peers; gathered basic information about AIDS and services; talked about powerless pasts; discussed sexual partners, dates, and lovers; developed political perspectives on homosexuality or their infections; and/or became politicized AIDS activists. Most learned the language and customs of recovery through 12-step support groups. Many saw therapists and relied on therapeutically versed friends. For many, their HIV status became the defining element in their lives, and their worlds came to revolve around partners, peers, and adults involved in AIDS-related work.

Many obtained employment in AIDS service or empowerment programs. Employment in empowerment programs was a source of self-esteem for many youths living with HIV and AIDS, providing normality, purpose, and a routine to often chaotic lives. Participation provided a much-needed source of income. However, significant paradoxes existed. Participation in empowerment programs allowed youths to financially survive for the present, but often did not encourage future *life empowerment*. To be successful in these programs, youths rapidly must move from client to provider roles, from *the helped* to *the helper*. They were expected to be peer role models. However, in their private lives and activities, youths often struggled with and engaged in many of the same risk activities that they were publicly working to prevent. Jack's behaviors were the most problematic example. This metamorphosis from client to provider was often impossible to accomplish and had significant negative consequences. Instead of being vehicles to the mainstream, participation in empowerment programs often caused many to feel inadequate and ill-prepared to work in professions other than AIDS-related ones. Youths often did not develop interpersonal skills employable in their own sexual lives or occupational skills that could be transferred to other jobs (Luna and Rotheram-Borus, 1997a). For many the work proved too stressful or consuming, and did not allow them to grow or realize ambitions. For some, it became stifling, unhelpful, even unhealthy.

The relationships between service program managers and youths as employees complicated an already challenging period, as there were unspoken expectations that peer educators, especially those living with HIV and AIDS, present a healthy, coping self to their peers and audiences. This shift from the client to the provider role, where adolescents or young adults must provide advice and an example for others, was not one that many were able to accomplish without anxiety. Their lives were increasingly regulated and ordered according to the empowerment ideology that characterized these programs. "Agreeable," "obedient," "capable," "together" behavior led to favorable status in the system. "Difficult," "argumentative," "self-destructive," "dysfunctional" behavior led to forcible expulsion, the termination of a work contract, or early "aging out." Some young people living with HIV were overwhelmed by the pressures of a service system and its' institutional empowerment ideology, which added to the burdens some youths carried in their private lives and public forums. Others lost their own support system while providing support for others. This was true for Jose and Jack. Many peer educators living with HIV or AIDS were unable to "practice what they preached," and they felt guilty as a result.

For empowered young people who lived troubled lives, HIV led to significant life changes and affected social functioning. Major life adaptations, reorganization, and behavioral changes followed. For less empowered youths, HIV was experienced as only another adverse life event without immediate consequence. They were experiencing other social problems. No life changes were considered immediately necessary, and behavioral routines and practices were continued. This was especially true for poor youths like Ethan and Mark who experienced more ongoing life crises (Rotheram-Borus et al., 1994), trauma, and poor hygienic living conditions. HIV infection was sometimes perceived by marginal or disenfranchised youths, such as Lisa, as beneficial, and facilitated easier access to social and health services and made available additional financial assistance and housing. Youths seeking services as clients (rather than those who served as employees) had opportunities to reject HIV identity, explore health alternatives derived from their cultures, and set respectful limits within the provider-client relationship.

For the troubled youths studied, their problems did not cease in childhood, but continued, overlapped, or even accelerated in adulthood as the result of earlier life experiences. Traumatic life events forced some to seek help or change the course of their lives. For others, such events led to further experimentation with a resulting desolation and vexation of spirit. Many youths were lured into exotic, erotic, narcotic misconduct in search of affection or stability, in self-harmful continuance of past traumas, or in existential search for meaning and personal relevance. They often became stuck in brief pleasures or favorite pastimes that were a hindrance to self-development or protective health behaviors. Some, like Jared, pursued bohemian lives where they misspent their youth. While still in their early and later teens, they did not necessarily have regrets. However, a few years later, in young adulthood, the realization that their lives lacked direction or purpose occurred, and this crisis encouraged important and necessary life changes. For some youths who lived with HIV and AIDS, such as Ethan, this crisis was ongoing, for others, such as Jared, it was acute.

For more affluent youths, HIV infection was often a more significant life event than for those youths from poor or disenfranchised backgrounds. Even though it was increasingly clear that HIV can be nonprogressive, youths planning extensive educational training or those having future aspirations and plans were forced to reevaluate their life goals, especially when T-cell counts dropped, viral activity increased, or HIV-related symptoms or problems occurred. Testing HIV positive initially induced depression, distress, anxiety, regrets, fear, and feelings of low self-worth.

The personal explanations and narratives of youths living with HIV reflect their behavioral and social adaptations, strategies employed, and coping actions following notification. They also illustrate youths' discovery, exploration, clarification, and consideration of past traumas. During and after interviews, many youths were better able to understand life events that led up to their HIV infections and the challenges that subsequently occurred. Many had never discussed the topics covered in interviews with anyone. They often found meaning in their recalled experiences. Patterns across narratives existed. For example, high-risk sexuality decreased or ended after HIV infection was diagnosed, and the need for social intimacy became greater. Paradoxically, this was also the time when most were isolated. For those who withheld the knowledge of their HIV status from others and avoided support services, life was particularly difficult and lonely.

Chapter 14

Conclusions

I draw in my wings. Happy me; I already breathe
freedom. I see it as a distant Alpine glow. Oh dawn!
To the ear it sounds like soft songs of victory. And
in the desert waste my voice resounds, like Mem-
non's column greeting the dawn.

—Karl Heinrich Ulrichs, *Memnon* (In Kennedy, 1988)

Sweet wizard, in whose footsteps I have trod
Unto the shrine of the most obscene god,
So steep the pathway is, I may not know,
Until I reach the summit, where I go.
My love is deathless as the springs of truth,
My love is pure as is the dawn of youth,
But all my being throbs in rhythm with thine,
Who leadest on to the horizon-line.

—Victor B. Neuburg, *The Triumph of Pan,* 1989

There were similar paths that the lives of youths living with HIV infection followed. Specific "life landmarks" or personally significant life events were identified through their narratives, as were recollections of past experiences, present activities, and adaptational strategies. Normal developmental exploration and risk taking were complicated by the environments in which developmental tasks were accomplished. Feelings from childhood were identical: Most felt unwanted, neglected, insecure, and unloved. All had been wounded early and had difficulties with attachments and relationships, and many were emotionally or physically transient. Most expressed same-sex preferences and had engaged in voluntary or involuntary nonprotective sexual activities. Others had long histories of shared intravenous drug use and substance addiction. Few maintained good relationships with their families; most were disenfranchised. All were articulate, most without benefit of much formal education. Many had run away or been thrown out of their homes, and many were clients of social service agencies. Some lived in poverty-ridden, drug-saturated, urban environments. These youths were street-smart, and many were self-supportive. Others used the system to their economic advantage to generate income and identify available options.

Life landmarks and specific experiences recalled by youths were necessary for creating explanatory stories. Explanatory infection stories were employed to represent how and why infection occurred, and gave personal and social meaning and relevance to the experience (Kleinman, 1980). Infection stories were necessary for accessing services, as well as for notifying family, friends, or future sexual partners of infection status. They were also used to corroborate or justify behaviors, as well as to develop a coherent version of their experiences. Through infection stories, some were able to reconcile "unforgivable" events that occurred in their pasts. However, most used "denial as defense" to avoid retrospection or introspection that could produce further distress or anxiety. The majority avoided contemplation of HIV-related issues until health failures made considerations unavoidable (Luna and Rotheram-Borus, 1997a; Luna and Rotheram-Borus, 1997b; Welle, Luna, and Rotheram-Borus, 1996c).

Similarities existed in the types of risk situations engaged in, including unprotected sex and shared-needle drug use, and in the toxic environments where they lived before and after infection. Suggestive findings connected to the four thematic areas explored can be summarized.

- Troubled familial or social backgrounds were present in the lives of the youths interviewed, regardless of social class or sexual preference. Parallel histories of physical and sexual abuse, emotional abandonment, and runaway behaviors were common. Intolerance and negative labeling connected to sexual preference or perceived inappropriateness of gender role performance often led to runaway behaviors.

- Most of the youths identified the specific individual or incident by which HIV infection occurred. All had created explanatory stories that included infection episodes. For the overwhelming majority of youths, highly intimate behaviors were not engaged in at first meeting, or without consideration with unknown strangers. Instead, they occurred after knowing and caring about partners over time, in order to please them, or in hope of solidifying otherwise unstable relationships. It must be emphasized that the majority of youths interviewed stated they were in "love" with the person they believe caused their HIV infection. In many instances, they were infected during their first sexual or love relationship. In most instances, infection occurred within "loving," "monogamous" relationships. Most of the youths studied knew of "safe sex precautions" prior to the time they believed they were infected. However, the specificity of knowledge varied greatly. Breaches and betrayals in trust were major factors that led to HIV infection. Joshua and Marie, for example, were intentionally deceived by infected partners. The interconnection with substance abuse cannot be minimized. Behavioral disinhibitions occurred as a result of substance use. A ritualistic character to shared needle use or the exchange of body fluids was also evident (Rotheram-Borus et al., 1994). The emotional and psychological reasons why some youths shared a death wish, or wanted to experience HIV with infected partners were complex (Rotheram-Borus et al., 1994). A romanticized desire to die along with the lover reflected as much on the present relationship, as on the more problematic features of their past relationships. All craved *real* affection and commitment.
- Most youths were connected to the social or health care system prior to testing HIV positive. Many had been long-term, difficult, "chronic" service clients and were well known to service providers. They often required long-term assistance, and given the obstacles that had to be overcome, drained the majority of the system's funds and resources. Many used or were used by the system (Luna and Rotheram-Borus, 1997a). Privacy and confidentiality were especially hard to manage for youths served in the system. Participation in support groups and inte-

grated health and social services often fostered involuntary disclosure. Notification was mishandled from the middle to later
1980s, with improvements made since 1992. Many youth were
unprepared for notification, and were traumatized by inap-
propriate behaviors or information given by providers.

• Posttest experiences varied, but can be grouped into four primary adaptational responses. For analytic purposes, four simple
adaptational stages can be identified, two reactive and two proactive. They are as follows: (1) anger, blame, or denial; (2) rejection, acting out, and self-harmful behaviors; (3) the creation of
infection stories, and search for information, assistance, and
acceptance; and finally, (4) the development of life-affirming
and future orientations (Luna and Rotheram-Borus, 1997c).
Readiness or unwillingness to accept service interventions varied. It must be understood that youths differed in their readiness to deal with HIV infection and to participate in structured
programs. Some were involved with HIV services only in
order to obtain scarce resources unavailable to alienated or disenfranchised youths without HIV infection. Social service
agencies routinely retested for HIV to screen out the increasing
numbers of youths who falsely claimed to be infected. Given
the long-term problems experienced by the youths studied, life
adjustments were slow and incremental. Self-harmful acts
including unprotected sex work and intravenous substance
usage were not totally discontinued, but with integrated and
comprehensive support services, such acts were often curtailed. However, the psychological underpinnings, motiva-
tions, and individual and societal reasons why these activities
were initially engaged in often went unidentified, and therefore
unaddressed. The economic rationale for high-risk sexual
behaviors can be addressed with housing, food supplements,
and General Assistance. However, youth with poor communication skills before testing HIV positive continued to maintain poor skills afterwards. Prior to HIV infection, many
youths lacked communication skills, other than those necessary to obtain scarce resources from providers. Some knew the
language of the streets, but lacked knowledge of the service
delivery system. In time, and within these contexts, they

learned what to say and do to get what they needed. However, after histories of abuse, most were unable to communicate their past troubles and feelings in ways that were self-protective. Their friends or service providers knew very little of their past or of their plans for the future. Whenever possible, they avoided situations where they felt vulnerable, situations that usually resulted in their victimization.

After lives filled with abuse and disenfranchisement, adaptation to HIV was of less significance than concerns over unemployment and the establishment and development of loving relationships with sexual partners. Cultural background and race, economic conditions and resources, family support, sexual orientation, age and experience, gender, pregnancy status, environment and housing, and relationship status (monogamous, dating, single) all affected adaptation to HIV to a greater or lesser degree. The significance of how notification was conducted and how youth eventually adapt to their HIV status, whether or not they were prepared correctly, and if it was traumatic cannot be underestimated. Notification of HIV infection was a major life event, and "testing positive" was always life altering even if not immediately stressful. The youths' social network was significant in encouraging and facilitating risk activities prior to and after infection and in the provision of subsequent support.

Sociability after notification of HIV infection generally decreased. Many youths were isolative after their status was determined, and contrary to popular beliefs, their sexual activities decreased sharply. These youths were not interactive and communicative after diagnosis. Others were unwilling or unable to participate in group activities requiring communication skills they previously lacked. Denial played an important role, especially for those youths otherwise prone to negative impulses or self-harmful behaviors. However, many continued in the same activities that led to their infection. For those youths who accepted their HIV status and engaged in HIV-support activities with others, reinfective behaviors were often hidden from service providers to avoid repercussions, including reductions or termination of support.

The implications are many. First and foremost, critical to addressing high-risk behaviors in youths is developing and fostering their interpersonal communication and negotiation skills. Underlying psychological states and conditions that influence if not determine future activities must subsequently be addressed. Low self-esteem and self-worth cause many youths to participate in high-risk, self-harmful acts because they believe they are not entitled to, or worthy of, better lives or treatment. Interventions that acknowledge and appreciate cultural diversity, enhance self-esteem, reward coopera-tion, and encourage positive relationships will promote the health and well-being of youths living with HIV. Pluralistic norms for socially competent coping behaviors are more likely to result in positive self-concepts, particularly for disenfranchised or sexual minority youth. Positive adaptation and coping can be fostered by developing interpersonal skills and abilities, and creating opportuni-ties for their use. Nonprogressive HIV and AIDS is now considered more of a chronic than immediately terminal disease. As a result, improvements in psychological status can be generated through *eco-nomic empowerment*, the development of career options, and future planning.

Interventions must consider and address the environmental and social contexts of risk behaviors and the personal management of drug use before and after infection. Relocation to less toxic environ-ments may be indicated (Rotheram-Borus et al., 1994). Situational, temporal, and developmental variation in risk behaviors exist, including differences based upon level of risk related to specific activities (anal receptive, oral receptive versus anal insertive, oral insertive). Competing risks must be considered and addressed. For example, most of the youths interviewed in service programs were career drug users, and they learned to manage their drug use. Less attention must be given to total cessation of substance use and more to encouraging moderation. Self-consciousness raising activities, which foster an understanding of the circumstances and situations wherein infection or reinfection occurs, are necessary. Family mem-bers, friends, or providers can help youths set, define, and opera-tionalize accomplishable, concrete, short- and long-term goals.

Explanatory models for understanding adaptation to HIV and for coping with disease progression need to be better understood and appreciated. Youths studied believed that when they began to con-centrate on their HIV infection, they would experience more illnesses and clinical symptomology of AIDS. These beliefs may have been related to adolescent denial and feelings of invincibility, or to drug-induced feelings of euphoria that precluded any sense of illness or "disease" until drug withdrawals when illness episodes were common (Carey and Mandel, 1968; Rotheram-Borus et al., 1994). Combination therapies or successful clinical trial "cocktails" with protease inhibitors, which decreased drops in T cells and caused less viral activity, were often described to youths with nonprogressive HIV to encourage them to enter therapeutic protocols immediately. Most resisted entry into protocols until substantial drops in their T cells occurred. An unwarranted sense of urgency was exacerbated by some health providers. A well-intentioned but unfounded sense of hope, which was not supported by proven clinical efficacy at the time, was encouraged, creating further dependency and subsequently, despair. When given a clear explanation of their options, most of the youths could understand and make informed decisions for their treatment.

Healthy behaviors, including dietary practices and personal hygiene (Marotta, 1996) must be encouraged, and self-help skills supported (Erskine and Judd, 1994). Exercise, spiritual development, and stress reduction can be effective ways to prolong the onset of AIDS. Massage, body work, biofeedback, and personally relevant religious or spiritual practices can all be beneficial (Welle, Luna, and Rotheram-Borus, 1996b). Personally meaningful rituals or "rites of passage" can be designed to promote developmental and spiritual growth and to help in coping with HIV (Welle, Luna, and Rotheram-Borus, 1996b). They also can help obtain closure on traumatic life events or aid in the transition from undesirable past social identities. Youths living with HIV can then proceed with their lives, putting past difficulties into perspective or to rest, and concentrating their efforts on more immediate or future life challenges.

Chapter 15

Afterward:
"Sail Forth to Seek and Find": Andy

Sleep, soldiers! still in honored rest
Your truth and valor wearing:
The bravest are the tenderest,–
The loving are the daring.

—Bayard Taylor, *The Poet's Journal,* 1863

I return for my wings,
let me return.
I want to die being
yesterday.
I want to die being
dawn.
I return for my wings,
let me return.
I want to die being
fountain.
I want to die away
from the sea.

—Federico Garcia Lorca, *Speech by a Raindrop*
(In Spender and Gili, 1939)

The life of one particular youth was especially memorable and compelling. His character and situation were similar to other disenfranchised youths or young adults infected with HIV in the 1980s, many of whom have died of AIDS.

Andy was thrown out of his New Jersey home in 1983 at age thirteen when his parents discovered that he had sex with a male classmate. He passed the majority of his early adolescence in institutions, running from foster home to foster home, and moving from city to city. Like other homeless youths in similar circumstances, he was involved in sexual activity for money, and sold and used a variety of drugs to support himself and to lessen his emotional pain. One specific, seemingly insignificant episode in his life proved particularly illustrative and was a metaphor for his character, situation, and general nature. It also marked a major turning point in his life passage.

By 1987, at age seventeen, Andy had been periodically "hustling" in San Francisco for eight months. He was supporting two younger street kids in a Tenderloin squat. He considered himself the head of a "family," and "sold himself" to keep others out of the street scene. He recalled at that time, he was picked up by a *trick* on Polk Street, a middle-aged physician, and was taken back to his house. Andy remembered that while there, he rummaged through a box of mostly pornographic tapes, and selected and played a video of the film *Now, Voyager*, featuring Bette Davis. He made this selection because he thought the title strange. Andy was immediately engaged, and empathized with the main character, who in the film from childhood through young adulthood had been thought an oddball—the clumsy, sensitive, unattractive member of the family. Andy related.

To others, especially the men who picked him up, Andy was confident and physically attractive. He never felt that way about himself. While watching the video, he said he recalled his own ambivalent sexual feelings, the emotional pull and concurrent fear of girls, his physical attraction to other boys, and his sense of loneliness and worthlessness. Andy had been physically and psychologically abused by his parents. He had never felt wanted, never unconditionally loved.

Ten minutes into the video, Andy remembered, the physician became amorous. Andy knew how to "work a trick," and was able to fend him off until after he finished watching the entire video. They had sex as agreed—Andy was paid, and he then left. Later, walking to the Castro Metro Station and feeling in his words "degraded and despondent," he passed the *Now, Voyager* Travel Agency on Eighteenth Street. He had passed by there many times before. However, he never paid attention to the name of the business. In further reflection on the film, he said he was particularly pleased that eventually the Davis character came into her own as a self-sufficient, independent person. The phrase used for the title of the film especially moved him, but he could not recall the exact words.

The following day, he went to the Public Library and asked a librarian for a book about or titled *Now, Voyager*. Andy thought that the "gay librarian" hesitated, and then appeared amused as he brought him Walt Whitman's book of poetry *Leaves of Grass*. He read carefully through almost the entire book before he returned to the "Passage to India" section. He copied the following, "*The untold want, by life and land ne'er granted, now, voyager, sail thou forth, to seek and find.*" That same week, he bought a used paperback copy of Whitman's poetry and learned that Whitman, like himself, had been homosexual. It was later learned that Andy loaned the book to many others for inspiration.

From then on, he always carried books of poetry or literature in his backpack. He would often quote from one book or another. He did not do this to impress people. He derived a sense of personal satisfaction and enjoyment from reading about utopian conditions or places; obvious contrasts to his own situation, and the life he lived. He planned on finishing his General Education Diploma, and dreamed of college. He said until his life changed, the streets would continue to be his "University."

Along with the books in his backpack were the simple, but significant artifacts of his transitory teenage street life: pictures of other street youth he had met, including male and female lovers, small bags of marijuana and speed, political flyers, a walkman radio, Guns and Roses cassette tapes, a toothbrush and toothpaste, and most significantly, letters and crayon drawings from a younger brother, still living at home, for whom he maintained affection and concern.

For three and one-half years from age eighteen, Andy was interviewed on a regular basis in San Francisco, at other times in Los Angeles, or San Diego. After short absences, he would appear at a youth agency or health clinic, write a postcard or periodically telephone collect to keep in contact. He was frequently involved in one political cause or another. For example, Andy organized a group of street youth to attend a Michael Dukakis speech during the 1988 Presidential Campaign. Governor Dukakis shook his hand, and

Andy slipped him a prepared list that outlined the service needs of street youth. He was disillusioned following the election and the Dukakis loss.

Andy was diagnosed with AIDS in 1989. He was sure he had been infected in his early teens through using tainted needles or having unprotected sex. He died of AIDS in 1992 in a public hospital following his twenty-second birthday. Given his situation, his past history, and lack of resources, his final acts were particularly inspirational and compelling: his willingness to share what little he had with others; his advocacy and volunteer work with street youths in shelters and agencies; and his early efforts in Act-Up and Queer Nation organizing street youths living with HIV and AIDS.

The best way to assist youths living with nonprogressive HIV, to help those with AIDS, or to honor those who have succumbed is to work toward rapid economic, political, social, and institutional change. Societies, communities, families, institutions, and services must be fostered wherein the troubled, disenfranchised, or marginalized are spared the abuse and degradations so often experienced. Adolescent experimentation, self-exploration, and characteristic altruism must be encouraged. On direct, interpersonal, and preventive levels, self-esteem, self-worth, and security must be nurtured within youths, enabling them to overcome childhood challenges, and confidently *sail forth to seek and find*.

Bibliography

Bond, L.S. (Ed.). *A portfolio of AIDS/STD behavioral interventions and research.* Washington, DC: Pan American Health Organization, 1992.

Brown, J., and Langley, J. Interviewer as instrument: Qualitative data collection and analysis using the principles of Gestalt and Confluent Education. Unpublished Paper. *Southwest Regional Laboratory*, 1991.

Carey, J.T., and Mandel, J. A San Francisco bay area "speed" scene. *Journal of Health and Social Behavior*, 9: 164-174, 1968.

Carpenter, E. (Ed.). *Iolaus: An anthology of friendship.* London: Swan Sonnenschein and Co., 1906.

Carpenter, E. *The intermediate sex: A study of transitional types of men and women.* London: Swan Sonnenschein and Co., 1909.

Carpenter, E. *Towards democracy.* New York: Mitchell Kennerley, 1912.

Cory, D.W. *The homosexual in America: A subjective approach.* New York: Greenberg, 1951.

Cory, D.W. *Homosexuality: A cross-cultural perspective.* New York: The Julian Press, Inc., 1956.

Cranston, K. HIV education for gay, lesbian, and bisexual youth: Personal risk, personal power, and the community of conscience. Special Issue: Coming out of the classroom closet. *Journal of Homosexuality*, 22(3-4): 247-259, 1991.

Dalven, R. (Trans.). *The complete poems of Cavafy.* New York: Harcourt, Brace and World, Inc., 1961.

Dover, K.J. *Greek homosexuality.* Cambridge, MA: Harvard University Press, 1978.

Edelstein, E.L., Nathanson, D.L., and Stone, A. (Eds.). *Denial: A clarification of concepts and research.* New York: Plenum Press, 1989.

Ellis, H., and Symonds, J.A. *Sexual inversion.* London: Wilson and Macmillan, 1897. (Reprint: New York: Arno Press, 1975).

Erskine, A., and Judd, D. (Eds.). *The imaginative body: Psychodynamic therapy in health care.* London, England: Whurr Publishers, Ltd., 1994.

Fremont-Smith, E. AIDS: Latest lit. *Village Voice*, August 16: 43-44, 1983.

Freud, S. *An outline of psycho-analysis.* Translated from the 1940 German edition by J. Strachey. New York: W.W. Norton & Co., 1949.

Garland, H. Roadside meetings of a literary nomad. *Bookman*, 70(December): 392-406, 1929.

Genet, J. *The thief's journal.* Translated from the 1949 French edition by Bernard Frechtman. Collection Merlin, Paris: The Olympia Press, 1954.

Gide, A. *Persephone.* Translated from the 1934 French Opera by Samuel Putnam. New York: The Gotham Book Mart, 1949.

Glaser, B., and Strauss, A. *The discovery of grounded theory: Strategies for qualitative research.* New York: Aldine Publishing, 1967.

Hooker, E. A preliminary analysis of group behavior of homosexuals. *Journal of Psychology*, 41: 217-225, 1956.

Humboldt, A. *Aspects of nature.* Translated from the 1849 third German edition by Mrs. Sabine (Two Volumes). London: Longman, Brown, Green, and Longmans; John Murray, Albermarle Street, 1849.

Humboldt, A. *Cosmos: A sketch of a physical description of the universe.* Translated from the 1844 German edition by E. C. Otte (Four Volumes). New York: Harper and Brothers Publishers, 1852.

Hunter, J., and Schaecher, R. AIDS prevention for lesbian, gay, and bisexual adolescents. Special Issue: HIV/AIDS. *Families in Society*, 75(6): 346-354, 1994.

Kennedy, H. *Ulrichs: The life and works of Karl Heinrich Ulrichs, pioneer of the modern gay movement.* Boston: Alyson Publications, Inc., 1988.

Kleinman, A. *Patients and healers in the context of culture: An exploration of the borderline between anthropology, medicine, and psychiatry.* Berkeley: University of California Press, 1980.

Langness, L.L., and Frank, G. *Lives: An anthropological approach to biography.* Novato, California: Chandler, Sharp Publishers, Inc., 1981.

Leyland, W. (Ed.). *Gay Sunshine interviews, volume one.* San Francisco: Gay Sunshine Press, 1978.

Leyland, W. (Ed.). *Gay Sunshine interviews, volume two.* San Francisco: Gay Sunshine Press, 1982.

Louys, P. (Trans.). *The songs of Bilitis.* Privately Printed: The Parnassian Society, 1920.

Luna, G.C. HIV and homeless youth. *Focus*, 2(10), 1987a, p. 3.

Luna, G.C. Welcome to my nightmare: The graffiti of homeless youth. *Society Magazine*, 24: 73-78, 1987b.

Luna, G.C. Street youth: Adaptation and survival in the AIDS decade. *J Adolescent Health,* 12(7): 497-582, 1991.

Luna, G.C. Working the john/servicing the client: Research and outreach on the "demand side" of male sex work. *CASH Newsletter*, 1(1): 8-9, 1994a.

Luna, G.C. Two perspectives on hustling. *CASH Newsletter*, 1(4): 10-11, 1994b.

Luna, G.C., Bond, L.S., and Zacarias, F. Implementing the Kingston Declaration: Behavioral interventions for preventing STDs and HIV in the Americas. In L.S. Bond (Ed.). *A Portfolio of AIDS/STD Behavioral Interventions and Research.* Washington, DC: Pan American Health Organization, 1992.

Luna, G.C., and Rotheram-Borus, M.J. Street youth and the AIDS Pandemic. Special Supplement. *AIDS Education and Prevention*, 4: 1-13, 1992.

Luna, G.C., and Rotheram-Borus, M.J. The limitations of empowerment programs for youth living with HIV. Department of Psychiatry, University of California, Los Angeles, 1997a (In submission).

Luna, G.C., and Rotheram-Borus, M.J. Youth living with HIV in the suburbs. Department of Psychiatry, University of California, Los Angeles, 1997b (In preparation).

Marotta, T. The wisdom of green cleaning: Ecological maintenance as preventive medicine. Unpublished manuscript. San Francisco: Green Cleaning Institute, 1996.

Martin, A.D., and Hetrick, E.S. The stigmatization of the gay and lesbian adolescent. *Journal of Homosexuality*, 15: 163-183, 1988.

Mills, C.W. *The sociological imagination*. New York: Oxford University Press, 1959.

Musil, R. *Young Torless*. Translated from the 1906 German edition by Eithne Wilkins and Ernst Kaiser. New York: Pantheon Books, 1955.

Neuburg, V. *The triumph of Pan*. London: Skoob Books Publishing Ltd., 1989.

Pater, W. *Miscellaneous studies: A series of essays*. London: Macmillan and Co., 1895.

Poppen, P.J., and Reisen, C.A. Heterosexual behaviors and risk of exposure to HIV: Current status and prospects for change. *Applied and Preventive Psychology*, 3 (2): 75-90, 1994.

Rimbaud, A. *A season in hell*. Translated from the 1873 French edition by Delmore Schwartz. Norfolk, CN: New Directions Books, 1939.

Rotheram-Borus, M.J., Luna, G.C., Marotta, M., and Kelly, H. Going nowhere fast: Methamphetamine use and HIV Infection. In R.J. Battjes, Z. Sloboda, and W.C. Grace (Eds.). *The context of HIV risk among drug users and their sexual partners*. NIDA Research Monograph 143, Rockville, MD: U.S. Department of Health and Human Services, 1994.

Rowse, A.L. *Homosexuals in history: Ambivalence in society, literature, and the arts*. New York: Macmillan Publishing Co., Inc., 1977.

Sarotte, G.M. *Like a brother, like a lover: Male homosexuality in the American novel and theater from Herman Melville to James Baldwin*. New York: Anchor Press/Doubleday, 1978.

Shakespeare, W. *The works of Shakespeare*. Volume the Seventh (*Troilus and Cressida*). London: Printed for J. and R. Tonfon et. al. , 1767.

Spender, S., and Gili, J.L. (Trans.). *Poems F. Garcia Lorca*. New York: Oxford University Press, 1939.

Steward, S.M. *Understanding the male hustler*. Binghamton, NY: Harrington Park Press, 1991.

Stoddard, C.W. *The lepers of Molokai*. Notre Dame, IN: The Ave Maria Press, 1910.

Strauss, A., and Corbin, J. *Basics of qualitative research*. Newbury Park, CA: Sage Publications, 1990.

Symonds, J.A. *Many moods: A volume of verse*. London: Smith, Elder, and Co., 1878.

Symonds, J.A. (Trans.). *The sonnets of Michael Angelo Buonarroti and Tommaso Campanella*. London: Smith, Elder, and Co., 1878.

Symonds, J.A. *A problem in modern ethics: Being an inquiry into the phenomenon of sexual inversion addressed especially to medical psychologists and jurists*. London: Privately Printed, 1896.

Swinburne, A.C. *Tristram of Lyonesse and other poems*. London: Chatto and Windus, Piccadilly, 1882.

Taylor, B. *The poet's journal*. Boston: Ticknor and Fields, 1863.

Trevelyan, R.C. (Trans.). *The idylls of Theocritus*. New York: Albert and Charles Boni, 1925.

Vasina, J. *Oral tradition: A study in historical methodology*. Translated by H.M. Wright. Chicago: Aldine Publishing Company, 1965.

Verlaine, P. Charles Husson. In D.W. Cory (Ed. and Trans.). *21 variations on a theme*. New York: Greenberg Publisher, 1953.

Weigall, A. *Sappho of Lesbos: Her life and time*. London: Thornton Butterworth, Limited, 1937.

Welle, D., Luna, G.C., and Rotheram-Borus, M.J. " 'I'd rather just be positive': Adolescent females' rejection of the client role as adaptation to HIV status." Department of Psychiatry, University of California, Los Angeles, 1996a (Unpublished manuscript).

Welle, D., Luna, G.C., and Rotheram-Borus, M.J. "The role of folk healing and spiritual practices in adolescent females' coping with HIV." Department of Psychiatry, University of California, Los Angeles, 1996b (Unpublished manuscript).

Welle, D., Luna, G.C., and Rotheram-Borus, M.J. " 'It's a lot of thoughts': The process of female adolescent's adjustment to HIV." Department of Psychiatry, University of California, Los Angeles, 1996c (Unpublished manuscript).

Whitman, W. *November boughs*. Philadelphia: David McKay, 1888.

Whitman, W. *Leaves of grass*. Philadelphia: David McKay, 1900.

Williams, T. *One arm and other stories*. Mount Vernon, NY: New Directions Books, 1948.

Williams, T. *In the winter of cities*. Norfolk, CN: New Directions Books, 1956.

Williams, T. *Androgyne, mon amour*. New York: New Directions Books, 1977.

Williams, T. *Collected stories*. New York: New Directions Books, 1985.

Index

Order Your Own Copy of
This Important Book for Your Personal Library!

YOUTHS LIVING WITH HIV
Self-Evident Truths

_____ in hardbound at $39.95 (ISBN: 0-7890-0176-4)

_____ in softbound at $14.95 (ISBN: 1-56023-904-2)

COST OF BOOKS _____	☐ **BILL ME LATER:** ($5 service charge will be added) (Bill-me option is good on US/Canada/Mexico orders only; not good to jobbers, wholesalers, or subscription agencies.)
OUTSIDE USA/CANADA/ MEXICO: ADD 20%_____	
POSTAGE & HANDLING_____ (US: $3.00 for first book & $1.25 for each additional book) Outside US: $4.75 for first book & $1.75 for each additional book)	☐ Check here if billing address is different from shipping address and attach purchase order and billing address information. Signature_____
SUBTOTAL_____	☐ **PAYMENT ENCLOSED: $**_____
IN CANADA: ADD 7% GST _____	☐ **PLEASE CHARGE TO MY CREDIT CARD.**
STATE TAX_____ (NY, OH & MN residents, please add appropriate local sales tax)	☐ Visa ☐ MasterCard ☐ AmEx ☐ Discover ☐ Diner's Club
	Account # _____
FINAL TOTAL_____ (If paying in Canadian funds, convert using the current exchange rate. UNESCO coupons welcome.)	Exp. Date _____ Signature _____

Prices in US dollars and subject to change without notice.

NAME _____

INSTITUTION _____

ADDRESS _____

CITY _____

STATE/ZIP _____

COUNTRY _____ COUNTY (NY residents only) _____

TEL _____ FAX _____

E-MAIL_____
May we use your e-mail address for confirmations and other types of information? ☐ Yes ☐ No

Order From Your Local Bookstore or Directly From
The Haworth Press, Inc.
10 Alice Street, Binghamton, New York 13904-1580 • USA
TELEPHONE: 1-800-HAWORTH (1-800-429-6784) / Outside US/Canada: (607) 722-5857
FAX: 1-800-895-0582 / Outside US/Canada: (607) 772-6362
E-mail: getinfo@haworth.com
PLEASE PHOTOCOPY THIS FORM FOR YOUR PERSONAL USE.

BOF96